THE DIABETES COOKBOOK

A COMPLETE 30 DAY MEAL PLAN FOR NEWLY DIAGNOSED

SHEILA MAYNARD

TABLE OF CONTENTS

Breakfast - Chia Seed Pudding with Tropical Fruits

Lunch - Quinoa and Black Bean Salad

Dinner - Stuffed Mushrooms with Spinach and Feta

Day 4

Breakfast - Southwest Egg and Avocado Bow

Lunch - Grilled Chicken and Vegetable Skewers

Dinner - Mexican Zucchini Casserole

Day 5

Breakfast - Almond Flour Banana Bread with Fresh Berries

Lunch - Lentil and Vegetable Curry

Dinner - Baked Salmon with Dill and Lemon

Day 6

Breakfast - Baked Cinnamon Apple Chips

Lunch - Cauliflower and Broccoli Gratin

Dinner - Beef and Vegetable Stew

Day 7

Breakfast - Nut and Seed Mix

Lunch - Mediterranean Chickpea Stew

Dinner - Chicken and Mushroom Quiche
with Whole Wheat Crust

Day 8

Breakfast - Raspberry and Almond Chia
Pudding

Lunch - Grilled Asparagus Spears with
Lemon Aioli

Dinner - Turkey and Vegetable Stir-Fry

Day 9

Breakfast - Blueberry and Spinach
Smoothie

Lunch - Quinoa Salad with Roasted
Vegetables

Dinner - Shrimp and Zucchini Noodles
Stir-Fry

Day 10

Breakfast - Banana Nut Oatmeal

Lunch - Spinach and Feta Stuffed
Chicken Breast

Dinner - Grilled Vegetable and Quinoa
Bowl

Day 11

Breakfast - Greek Yogurt Parfait with Berries and Granola

Lunch - Quinoa and Avocado Salad

Dinner - Baked Cod with Lemon and Herbs

Day 12

Breakfast - Mixed Berry Smoothie Bowl

Lunch - Quinoa and Avocado Salad

Dinner - Baked Chicken with Roasted Vegetables

Day 13

Breakfast - Coconut and Mango Chia Pudding

Lunch - Quinoa and Black Bean Stuffed Bell Peppers

Dinner - Vegetable and Tofu Stir-Fry

Day 14

Breakfast - Chocolate Banana Protein Smoothie

Lunch - Mediterranean Quinoa Salad

Dinner - Salmon with Lemon Dill Sauce and Steamed Vegetables

Day 15

Breakfast - Apple Cinnamon Overnight Oats

Lunch - Caprese Salad with Balsamic Glaze

Dinner - Eggplant Parmesan with Marinara Sauce

Day 16

Breakfast - Veggie Omelette

Lunch - Chicken and Avocado Wrap

Dinner - Stir-Fried Tofu with Broccoli and Cashews

Day 17

Breakfast - Peanut Butter and Banana Toast

Lunch - Lentil and Vegetable Soup

Dinner - Shrimp and Asparagus Stir-Fry:

Day 18

Breakfast - Blueberry Almond Overnight Oats:

Lunch - Quinoa and Chickpea Salad

Dinner - Baked Turkey Meatballs with Zucchini Noodles

Day 19

Breakfast - Greek Yogurt and Berry
Parfait

Lunch - Spinach and Quinoa Stuffed Bell
Peppers

Dinner - Baked Cod with Lemon Garlic
Butter

Day 20

Breakfast - Green Smoothie Bowl:

Lunch - Turkey and Avocado Wrap

Dinner - Quinoa Stuffed Bell Peppers
with Black Beans

Day 21

Breakfast - Raspberry Chia Seed
Pudding

Lunch - Shrimp and Avocado Salad

Dinner - Baked Chicken and Vegetable
Foil Packets

Day 22

Breakfast - Almond Butter and Banana
Toast

Lunch - Lentil and Kale Soup

INTRODUCTION

Once upon a time, in a small town nestled among rolling hills, lived a remarkable woman named Isabella. She was an epitome of strength, and her spirit illuminated the lives of everyone she encountered. Isabella was diagnosed with diabetes at a young age, but she refused to let it define her.

Her kitchen was a haven of warmth and love, where she would whip up culinary delights that seemed to hold the power to heal not only the body but also the soul. Every dish that came from her stove was sprinkled with a dash of passion and a pinch of determination, each one a testament to her unyielding spirit.

One chilly winter evening, the town was buzzing with excitement as they prepared for the annual holiday feast. Isabella, being the heart and soul of the festivities, took it upon herself to create a menu that would make this year's celebration unforgettable. She decided to share her most cherished family recipes, ones that had been passed down for generations.

As the townsfolk gathered at the community hall, the air filled with a delectable aroma that seemed to dance around their senses. With each dish that emerged from the kitchen, Isabella would take center stage and narrate the story behind it. She spoke of her grandmother, who had instilled in her the love for cooking and the importance of embracing life's challenges with a smile.

One particular dish, a sumptuous vegetable stew, held a special significance. Isabella shared how it was her go-to comfort food during challenging times with diabetes. "Life is like this stew," she said with a twinkle in her eye, "It may have a mix of different flavors and experiences, but when we let them simmer together with patience and resilience, the result is a beautiful tapestry of taste and life lessons."

As the evening unfolded, Isabella's tales intertwined with the mouthwatering recipes, evoking laughter, tears, and a newfound appreciation for the strength within each person present. The sense of community grew stronger, and the invisible walls that had separated them seemed to crumble away, leaving behind a sense of unity and understanding.

Her cookbook, born from this magical night, became a timeless treasure passed on to generations. It wasn't just a collection of recipes; it was a living testament to the power of stories and the resilience of the human spirit. People from all walks of life, diabetics and non-diabetics alike, found solace, encouragement, and inspiration within its pages.

Isabella's legacy lived on, not only in her recipes but in the hearts of those who were touched by her indomitable spirit. Through the cookbook, she continued to weave her stories into the lives of countless others, reminding them that life's challenges can be transformed into triumphs with love, hope, and the magic of storytelling. And so, the little town embraced the diabetic cookbook, not only as a guide to delicious meals but as a celebration of life itself, sprinkled with the enchanting essence of Isabella's enduring spirit.

Day 1:

Breakfast - Greek Yogurt Breakfast Bowl with Berries and Nuts:

Ingredients:

- 1 cup Greek yogurt

- 1/2 cup mixed berries (strawberries, blueberries, raspberries)

- 2 tablespoons chopped nuts (almonds, walnuts, or pecans)

- 1 teaspoon honey (optional, for added sweetness)

Preparation:

1. In a bowl, add Greek yogurt as the base.

2. Top it with the mixed berries and chopped nuts.

3. Drizzle honey on top if desired.

4. Mix well and enjoy the wholesome and protein-packed breakfast.

Lunch - Turkey Lettuce Wraps with Avocado:

Ingredients:

- 4 large lettuce leaves (butter or romaine lettuce works well)
- 8 ounces cooked and sliced turkey breast
- 1 ripe avocado, sliced
- 1/2 cup diced tomatoes
- 1/4 cup diced red onion
- 1 tablespoon lime juice
- Salt and pepper to taste.

Preparation:

1. Lay the lettuce leaves flat on a plate.

2. Layer the sliced turkey, avocado, diced tomatoes, and red onion on each lettuce leaf.

3. Drizzle lime juice over the toppings and season with salt and pepper.

4. Roll up the lettuce leaves to create wraps.

5. Secure with toothpicks if needed, and serve these refreshing and satisfying lettuce wraps.

Dinner - Baked Herb-Crusted Chicken with Roasted Brussels Sprouts:

Ingredients:

- 2 boneless, skinless chicken breasts

- 1 tablespoon olive oil

- 1 teaspoon dried thyme

- 1 teaspoon dried rosemary

- 1 teaspoon dried oregano

- 1/2 teaspoon garlic powder

- 1/2 teaspoon onion powder

- Salt and pepper to taste

- 1 pound Brussels sprouts, trimmed and halved

Preparation:

1. Preheat the oven to 400°F (200°C).

2. Rub the chicken breasts with olive oil and season with dried thyme, rosemary, oregano, garlic powder, onion powder, salt, and pepper.

3. Place the seasoned chicken breasts on a baking sheet lined with parchment paper.

4. In a separate bowl, toss the halved Brussels sprouts with olive oil, salt, and pepper.

5. Arrange the Brussels sprouts on the same baking sheet around the chicken breasts.

6. Bake in the preheated oven for about 20-25 minutes or until the chicken is cooked through and the Brussels sprouts are roasted and tender.

7. Serve the herb-crusted chicken with a side of roasted Brussels sprouts for a delicious and nutritious dinner.

Day 2:

Breakfast - Low-carb Pancakes with Sugar-Free Maple Syrup:

Ingredients:

- 1 cup almond flour

- 2 tablespoons coconut flour

- 1 teaspoon baking powder

- 1/4 teaspoon salt

- 2 large eggs

- 1/4 cup unsweetened almond milk (or any milk of choice)

- 1 tablespoon melted butter or coconut oil

- Sugar-free maple syrup for topping

Preparation:

1. In a mixing bowl, whisk together almond flour, coconut flour, baking powder, and salt.

2. In a separate bowl, beat the eggs and mix in almond milk and melted butter or coconut oil.

3. Combine the wet and dry ingredients to form a pancake batter.

4. Heat a non-stick pan over medium heat and lightly grease it with cooking spray or butter.

5. Pour about 1/4 cup of the batter onto the pan to form each pancake.

6. Cook until bubbles appear on the surface, then flip and cook the other side until golden brown.

7. Serve the low-carb pancakes with sugar-free maple syrup for a delightful breakfast.

Lunch - Chickpea and Spinach Curry:

Ingredients:

- 1 can (15 ounces) chickpeas, drained and rinsed
- 1 tablespoon vegetable oil
- 1 large onion, finely chopped
- 2 cloves garlic, minced
- 1 tablespoon grated ginger
- 1 tablespoon curry powder
- 1 teaspoon ground cumin
- 1 teaspoon ground coriander
- 1/2 teaspoon turmeric powder
- 1 can (14 ounces) diced tomatoes
- 1 cup vegetable broth
- 2 cups fresh spinach leaves
- Salt and pepper to taste
- Fresh cilantro for garnish

Preparation:

1. In a large skillet, heat vegetable oil over medium heat.

2. Add chopped onions and cook until they become translucent.

3. Stir in minced garlic and grated ginger, sauté for another minute.

4. Add curry powder, cumin, coriander, and turmeric. Cook for a minute to release the flavors.

5. Pour in diced tomatoes and vegetable broth. Bring to a simmer.

6. Add chickpeas and let it simmer for 10 minutes to allow the flavors to meld.

7. Stir in fresh spinach leaves and cook until they wilt.

8. Season with salt and pepper to taste.

9. Garnish with fresh cilantro and serve the chickpea and spinach curry with brown rice or quinoa.

Dinner - Lemon-Garlic Grilled Fish with Cauliflower Rice Pilaf:

Ingredients:

- 2 white fish fillets (such as tilapia or cod)

- 2 tablespoons olive oil

- Zest and juice of 1 lemon

- 2 cloves garlic, minced

- Salt and pepper to taste

- 1 head cauliflower, grated or finely chopped

- 1/4 cup diced bell peppers

- 1/4 cup diced carrots

- 1/4 cup frozen peas

- 1 tablespoon chopped fresh parsley

Preparation:

1. In a shallow dish, combine olive oil, lemon zest, lemon juice, minced garlic, salt, and pepper.

2. Marinate the fish fillets in the lemon-garlic mixture for about 15 minutes.

3. Preheat the grill to medium-high heat. Grill the fish fillets for 3-4 minutes on each side or until cooked through.

4. For the cauliflower rice pilaf, heat a tablespoon of olive oil in a skillet over medium heat.

5. Add diced bell peppers, carrots, and frozen peas. Sauté for a few minutes until the vegetables are tender.

6. Stir in the grated cauliflower and cook for an additional 3-4 minutes until the cauliflower is cooked but still firm.

7. Season the cauliflower rice pilaf with salt, pepper, and chopped fresh parsley.

8. Serve the lemon-garlic grilled fish over the cauliflower rice pilaf for a light and flavorful dinner.

Day 3:

Breakfast - Chia Seed Pudding with Tropical Fruits:

Ingredients:

- 1/4 cup chia seeds

- 1 cup unsweetened coconut milk (or any milk of choice)

- 1 tablespoon honey or maple syrup (optional, for added sweetness)

- 1/2 cup diced tropical fruits (mango, pineapple, papaya)

- 1 tablespoon shredded coconut (unsweetened)

Preparation:

1. In a bowl, mix chia seeds with unsweetened coconut milk.

2. Add honey or maple syrup if desired for sweetness and stir well.

3. Cover the bowl and refrigerate for at least 4 hours or overnight to allow the chia seeds to absorb the liquid and form a pudding-like consistency.

4. Before serving, give the chia seed pudding a good stir.

5. Top the chia seed pudding with diced tropical fruits and shredded coconut for a refreshing and nutrient-packed breakfast.

Lunch - Quinoa and Black Bean Salad:

Ingredients:

- 1 cup cooked quinoa (follow package instructions)
- 1 can (15 ounces) black beans, drained and rinsed
- 1 cup diced cucumber
- 1 cup diced tomatoes
- 1/4 cup chopped red onion
- 1/4 cup chopped fresh cilantro
- 2 tablespoons lime juice
- 2 tablespoons olive oil
- Salt and pepper to taste

Preparation:

1. In a large bowl, combine cooked quinoa, black beans, diced cucumber, diced tomatoes, chopped red onion, and fresh cilantro.

2. In a separate bowl, whisk together lime juice, olive oil, salt, and pepper to make the dressing.

3. Pour the dressing over the quinoa and black bean mixture.

4. Toss well to coat all the ingredients with the dressing.

5. Refrigerate for 30 minutes to allow the flavors to meld.

6. Serve the quinoa and black bean salad chilled for a healthy and hearty lunch.

Dinner - Stuffed Mushrooms with Spinach and Feta:

Ingredients:

- 8 large button mushrooms

- 2 cups fresh spinach, chopped

- 1/4 cup crumbled feta cheese

- 2 cloves garlic, minced

- 1 tablespoon olive oil

- Salt and pepper to taste

Preparation:

1. Preheat the oven to 375°F (190°C).

2. Remove the stems from the mushrooms and carefully scoop out some of the gills to create space for the filling.

3. In a skillet, heat olive oil over medium heat.

4. Add minced garlic and sauté until fragrant.

5. Add chopped spinach to the skillet and cook until wilted.

6. Season with salt and pepper to taste.

7. Stuff each mushroom cap with the spinach mixture and top with crumbled feta cheese.

8. Place the stuffed mushrooms on a baking sheet and bake in the preheated oven for about 15 minutes or until the mushrooms are tender and the cheese is melted and lightly browned.

9. Serve the stuffed mushrooms as a delectable and nutritious dinner.

Day 4:

Breakfast - Southwest Egg and Avocado Bowl

Ingredients

- 1/4 cup black beans, drained and rinsed
- 1/4 cup diced tomatoes
- 1/4 cup diced bell peppers (red, green, or yellow)
- 1 tablespoon chopped fresh cilantro
- 1 tablespoon lime juice
- Salt and pepper to taste
- Hot sauce or salsa for extra flavor (optional)

Preparation:

1. Preheat the oven to 375°F (190°C).

2. Scoop out a small portion from the center of each avocado half to create a well for the egg.

3. Place the avocado halves in a baking dish to stabilize them.

4. Crack one egg into each avocado half, ensuring the yolk is intact.

5. Season the eggs with salt and pepper.

6. Bake in the preheated oven for about 12-15 minutes or until the eggs are cooked to your desired level of doneness.

7. While the eggs are baking, mix together black beans, diced tomatoes, diced bell peppers, chopped cilantro, lime juice, salt, and pepper in a bowl to create the salsa topping.

8. Once the eggs are cooked, remove the avocado halves from the oven and top each with the salsa mixture.

9. Drizzle with hot sauce or salsa for an extra kick, if desired.

10. Enjoy this southwestern-inspired breakfast with the creamy avocado and perfectly cooked eggs.

Lunch - Grilled Chicken and Vegetable Skewers:

Ingredients:

- 8 ounces boneless, skinless chicken breast, cut into bite-sized pieces
- 1 cup cherry tomatoes
- 1 cup zucchini chunks
- 1 cup bell pepper chunks (red, green, or yellow)
- 1 tablespoon olive oil
- 1 tablespoon lemon juice
- 1 teaspoon dried oregano

- 1 teaspoon dried thyme

- Salt and pepper to taste

Preparation:

1. Preheat the grill or grill pan over medium-high heat.

2. In a bowl, mix olive oil, lemon juice, dried oregano, dried thyme, salt, and pepper to create the marinade.

3. Thread the chicken pieces and vegetable chunks onto skewers, alternating between them.

4. Brush the chicken and vegetables with the marinade to coat them evenly.

5. Grill the skewers for about 10-12 minutes, turning occasionally, until the chicken is cooked through and the vegetables are charred and tender.

6. Remove the skewers from the grill and serve these delightful grilled chicken and vegetable skewers for a satisfying lunch.

Dinner - Mexican Zucchini Casserole:

Ingredients:

- 2 medium zucchinis, thinly sliced
- 1 cup cooked quinoa
- 1 can (15 ounces) black beans, drained and rinsed
- 1 cup diced tomatoes
- 1 cup diced bell peppers (red, green, or yellow)
- 1/2 cup diced red onion
- 1 tablespoon chili powder
- 1 teaspoon ground cumin
- 1/2 teaspoon garlic powder
- 1/2 teaspoon paprika
- 1/2 cup shredded cheddar cheese (reduced-fat if preferred)
- Fresh cilantro for garnish

Preparation:

1. Preheat the oven to 375°F (190°C).

2. In a large mixing bowl, combine sliced zucchinis, cooked quinoa, black beans, diced tomatoes, diced bell peppers, and diced red onion.

3. Add chili powder, ground cumin, garlic powder, and paprika. Mix well to coat the ingredients with the spices.

4. Transfer the mixture to a casserole dish and spread it out evenly.

5. Sprinkle shredded cheddar cheese over the top of the casserole.

6. Cover the casserole dish with foil and bake in the preheated oven for about 25-30 minutes or until the zucchinis are tender and the cheese is melted and bubbly.

7. Remove the foil and bake for an additional 5 minutes to lightly brown the cheese.

8. Garnish with fresh cilantro before serving this flavorful Mexican zucchini casserole for dinner.

Day 5:

Breakfast - Almond Flour Banana Bread with Fresh Berries:

Ingredients:

- 2 ripe bananas, mashed

- 2 large eggs

- 1/4 cup unsweetened applesauce

- 1 teaspoon vanilla extract

- 2 cups almond flour

- 1 teaspoon baking powder

- 1/2 teaspoon baking soda

- 1/2 teaspoon ground cinnamon

- 1/4 teaspoon salt

- 1/2 cup fresh berries (blueberries, raspberries, or strawberries)

Preparation:

1. Preheat the oven to 350°F (175°C). Grease a loaf pan and line it with parchment paper for easy removal.

2. In a large bowl, whisk together mashed bananas, eggs, unsweetened applesauce, and vanilla extract until well combined.

3. In a separate bowl, mix almond flour, baking powder, baking soda, ground cinnamon, and salt.

4. Gradually add the dry ingredients to the wet ingredients, stirring until just combined.

5. Gently fold in fresh berries into the batter.

6. Pour the batter into the prepared loaf pan, smoothing the top with a spatula.

7. Bake in the preheated oven for about 40-45 minutes or until a toothpick inserted into the center comes out clean.

8. Allow the almond flour banana bread to cool in the pan for 10 minutes, then transfer it to a wire rack to cool completely.

9. Slice and serve the banana bread with a side of fresh berries for a scrumptious and nutritious breakfast.

Lunch - Lentil and Vegetable Curry:

Ingredients:

- 1 cup dried red lentils

- 2 cups vegetable broth

- 1 can (14 ounces) diced tomatoes

- 1 cup diced carrots

- 1 cup diced zucchini

- 1 cup diced bell peppers (red, green, or yellow)

- 1 tablespoon vegetable oil

- 1 large onion, finely chopped

- 2 cloves garlic, minced

- 1 tablespoon grated ginger

- 2 tablespoons curry powder

- 1 teaspoon ground cumin

- 1 teaspoon ground coriander

- 1/2 teaspoon turmeric powder

- 1/2 cup coconut milk (unsweetened)

- Fresh cilantro for garnish

- Cooked brown rice or quinoa for serving

Preparation:

1. Rinse the red lentils under cold water and drain well.

2. In a large pot, heat vegetable oil over medium heat.

3. Add chopped onions and cook until they become translucent.

4. Stir in minced garlic and grated ginger, sauté for another minute.

5. Add curry powder, cumin, coriander, and turmeric. Cook for a minute to release the flavors.

6. Pour in vegetable broth and diced tomatoes, bring to a simmer.

7. Add diced carrots, zucchini, and bell peppers to the pot and let it simmer for 10 minutes to cook the vegetables.

8. Add the rinsed lentils to the pot and stir well.

9. Cover and simmer for about 15-20 minutes or until the lentils are tender and cooked through.

10. Stir in coconut milk to add creaminess to the curry.

11. Let the curry simmer for another 5 minutes to allow the flavors to meld together.

12. Season with salt and pepper to taste.

13. Garnish the lentil and vegetable curry with fresh cilantro.

14. Serve the flavorful and nutritious curry over cooked brown rice or quinoa for a satisfying lunch.

Dinner - Baked Salmon with Dill and Lemon:

Ingredients:

- 2 salmon fillets (about 6 ounces each)

- 1 tablespoon olive oil

- Zest and juice of 1 lemon

- 2 cloves garlic, minced

- 1 tablespoon chopped fresh dill

- Salt and pepper to taste

- Lemon slices for garnish

Preparation:

1. Preheat the oven to 375°F (190°C). Grease a baking dish or line it with parchment paper.

2. In a small bowl, whisk together olive oil, lemon zest, lemon juice, minced garlic, chopped dill, salt, and pepper to create the marinade.

3. Place the salmon fillets in the baking dish, skin-side down.

4. Pour the marinade over the salmon, making sure it is evenly coated.

5. Arrange lemon slices on top of the salmon fillets for extra flavor.

6. Cover the baking dish with foil and bake in the preheated oven for about 15-20 minutes or until the salmon is cooked through and easily flakes with a fork.

7. Remove the foil and bake for an additional 5 minutes to lightly brown the top.

8. Serve the baked salmon with dill and lemon with a side of roasted vegetables or a green salad for a delightful dinner.

Please note that the recipes provided are intended for individuals with diabetes, but it's essential to adjust portion sizes and ingredients as needed to fit individual dietary requirements and preferences. Always consult with a healthcare professional or a registered dietitian for personalized guidance on managing diabetes through diet.

Day 6:

Breakfast - Baked Cinnamon Apple Chips:

Ingredients:

- 2 large apples (Granny Smith or Honeycrisp), thinly sliced
- 1 tablespoon lemon juice
- 1 teaspoon ground cinnamon
- 1 tablespoon granulated sugar or sugar substitute (optional)

Preparation:

1. Preheat the oven to 225°F (110°C). Line a baking sheet with parchment paper.

2. In a bowl, toss the thinly sliced apples with lemon juice to prevent browning.

3. In a separate bowl, mix ground cinnamon and granulated sugar (if using).

4. Sprinkle the cinnamon mixture evenly over the apple slices and gently toss to coat.

5. Arrange the coated apple slices in a single layer on the prepared baking sheet.

6. Bake in the preheated oven for about 2 to 2.5 hours, flipping the slices halfway through, until they are crisp and slightly golden.

7. Allow the baked cinnamon apple chips to cool completely before enjoying this healthy and crunchy breakfast.

Lunch - Cauliflower and Broccoli Gratin:

Ingredients:

- 1 medium cauliflower head, cut into florets

- 1 medium broccoli head, cut into florets

- 1 cup shredded cheddar cheese (reduced-fat if preferred)

- 1 cup heavy cream or unsweetened almond milk

- 2 tablespoons unsalted butter

- 2 tablespoons all-purpose flour (or gluten-free flour)

- 1/2 teaspoon garlic powder

- 1/2 teaspoon onion powder

- Salt and pepper to taste

- Fresh parsley for garnish

Preparation:

1. Preheat the oven to 375°F (190°C). Grease a baking dish.

2. In a large pot of boiling salted water, blanch cauliflower and broccoli florets for 3-4 minutes until slightly tender. Drain and set aside.

3. In a separate saucepan, melt butter over medium heat.

4. Stir in flour and cook for about 1 minute to form a roux.

5. Slowly whisk in heavy cream or unsweetened almond milk, stirring continuously until the mixture thickens and becomes smooth.

6. Add garlic powder, onion powder, salt, and pepper to the sauce, and continue to stir until well combined.

7. Remove the saucepan from heat and stir in shredded cheddar cheese until it melts into the sauce.

8. In the prepared baking dish, layer blanched cauliflower and broccoli.

9. Pour the cheese sauce over the vegetables, ensuring they are evenly coated.

10. Bake in the preheated oven for about 20-25 minutes or until the gratin is bubbling and lightly golden on top.

11. Garnish with fresh parsley before serving this creamy and comforting cauliflower and broccoli gratin for lunch.

Dinner - Beef and Vegetable Stew:

Ingredients:

- 1 pound beef stew meat, cut into bite-sized pieces
- 1 tablespoon vegetable oil
- 1 large onion, chopped
- 2 cloves garlic, minced
- 2 medium carrots, sliced

- 2 medium potatoes, peeled and diced

- 1 cup diced tomatoes

- 4 cups beef broth (low-sodium if preferred)

- 1 tablespoon tomato paste

- 1 teaspoon dried thyme

- 1 bay leaf

- Salt and pepper to taste

- Fresh parsley for garnish

Preparation:

1. In a large pot or Dutch oven, heat vegetable oil over medium-high heat.

2. Add the beef stew meat and brown on all sides. Remove the beef from the pot and set aside.

3. In the same pot, sauté chopped onions until they become translucent.

4. Add minced garlic and cook for another minute.

5. Stir in sliced carrots, diced potatoes, and diced tomatoes.

6. Return the browned beef to the pot.

7. Pour in beef broth and add tomato paste, dried thyme, bay leaf, salt, and pepper.

8. Bring the stew to a boil, then reduce the heat to low, cover, and simmer for about 1.5 to 2 hours or until the beef is tender and the vegetables are cooked through.

9. Remove the bay leaf before serving.

10. Garnish with fresh parsley and enjoy this hearty and warming beef and vegetable stew for dinner.

Day 7:

Breakfast - Nut and Seed Mix:

Ingredients:

- 1/4 cup almonds

- 1/4 cup walnuts

- 1/4 cup pumpkin seeds

- 1/4 cup sunflower seeds

- 1/4 cup unsweetened coconut flakes

- 1/4 teaspoon ground cinnamon

- 1/4 teaspoon salt

Preparation:

1. In a bowl, combine almonds, walnuts, pumpkin seeds, sunflower seeds, and unsweetened coconut flakes.

2. Sprinkle ground cinnamon and salt over the nut and seed mixture.

3. Toss the ingredients together until the nuts and seeds are evenly coated with the cinnamon and salt.

4. Transfer the nut and seed mix to an airtight container for storage.

5. Serve this nutritious and crunchy nut and seed mix as a quick and satisfying breakfast option. You can also sprinkle it over yogurt or add it to smoothies for an extra boost of flavor and nutrients.

Lunch - Mediterranean Chickpea Stew:

Ingredients:

- 1 can (15 ounces) chickpeas, drained and rinsed
- 1 tablespoon olive oil
- 1 large onion, finely chopped
- 2 cloves garlic, minced
- 1 cup diced tomatoes
- 1 cup vegetable broth
- 1/2 cup pitted Kalamata olives, halved
- 1/4 cup chopped sun-dried tomatoes
- 1 teaspoon dried oregano
- 1 teaspoon dried basil
- Salt and pepper to taste
- Crumbled feta cheese for garnish
- Fresh parsley for garnish

Preparation:

1. In a large skillet, heat olive oil over medium heat.

2. Add chopped onions and cook until they become translucent.

3. Stir in minced garlic and cook for another minute.

4. Add diced tomatoes and vegetable broth. Bring to a simmer.

5. Add chickpeas, Kalamata olives, chopped sun-dried tomatoes, dried oregano, dried basil, salt, and pepper to the skillet.

6. Simmer for about 10-15 minutes to allow the flavors to meld together and the stew to thicken slightly.

7. Adjust seasoning if needed.

8. Garnish with crumbled feta cheese and fresh parsley before serving this delicious and Mediterranean-inspired chickpea stew for lunch.

Dinner - Chicken and Mushroom Quiche with Whole Wheat Crust:

Ingredients for Whole Wheat Crust:

- 1 cup whole wheat flour

- 1/4 teaspoon salt

- 1/4 cup unsalted butter, cold and cut into small cubes

- 3-4 tablespoons ice-cold water

Preparation for Whole Wheat Crust:

1. In a mixing bowl, whisk together whole wheat flour and salt.

2. Add cold butter cubes to the flour mixture.

3. Use a pastry cutter or fork to cut the butter into the flour until the mixture resembles coarse crumbs.

4. Gradually add ice-cold water, one tablespoon at a time, and mix until the dough comes together.

5. Shape the dough into a ball, wrap it in plastic wrap, and refrigerate for at least 30 minutes before rolling it out.

Ingredients for Chicken and Mushroom Quiche:

- Whole wheat crust (prepared as above)

- 1 cup cooked and shredded chicken breast

- 1 cup sliced mushrooms

- 1 cup baby spinach leaves

- 1/2 cup shredded cheddar cheese (reduced-fat if preferred)

- 4 large eggs

- 1 cup milk (whole, reduced-fat, or plant-based)

- Salt and pepper to taste

Preparation for Chicken and Mushroom Quiche:

1. Preheat the oven to 375°F (190°C). Grease a 9-inch pie dish.

2. On a lightly floured surface, roll out the chilled whole wheat crust to fit the pie dish.

3. Gently press the crust into the pie dish and trim any excess dough from the edges.

4. In a skillet, sauté sliced mushrooms until they release their moisture and become slightly browned.

5. In a separate bowl, whisk together eggs, milk, salt, and pepper to create the quiche filling.

6. Layer shredded chicken, sautéed mushrooms, and baby spinach leaves in the pie crust.

7. Pour the egg and milk mixture over the filling in the pie crust.

8. Sprinkle shredded cheddar cheese over the top.

9. Bake the quiche in the preheated oven for about 30-35 minutes or until the filling is set and the crust is golden brown.

10. Allow the quiche to cool slightly before slicing and serving this savory and satisfying chicken and mushroom quiche for dinner.

Day 8:

Breakfast - Raspberry and Almond Chia Pudding:

Ingredients:

- 1/4 cup chia seeds

- 1 cup unsweetened almond milk (or any milk of choice)

- 1 tablespoon honey or maple syrup (optional, for added sweetness)

- 1/2 cup fresh raspberries

- 1 tablespoon sliced almonds

Preparation:

1. In a bowl, mix chia seeds with unsweetened almond milk.

2. Add honey or maple syrup if desired for sweetness and stir well.

3. Cover the bowl and refrigerate for at least 4 hours or overnight to allow the chia seeds to absorb the liquid and form a pudding-like consistency.

4. Before serving, give the chia seed pudding a good stir.

5. Top the chia seed pudding with fresh raspberries and sliced almonds for a delightful and antioxidant-rich breakfast.

Lunch - Grilled Asparagus Spears with Lemon Aioli:

Ingredients:

- 1 bunch asparagus spears, tough ends trimmed

- 1 tablespoon olive oil

- Salt and pepper to taste

For Lemon Aioli:

- 1/4 cup mayonnaise (regular or light)

- Zest and juice of 1 lemon

- 1 clove garlic, minced

- Salt and pepper to taste

Preparation:

1. Preheat the grill or grill pan over medium-high heat.

2. Toss asparagus spears with olive oil, salt, and pepper until they are evenly coated.

3. Grill the asparagus spears for about 5-7 minutes, turning occasionally, until they are lightly charred and tender.

4. In a small bowl, whisk together mayonnaise, lemon zest, lemon juice, minced garlic, salt, and pepper to make the lemon aioli sauce.

5. Serve the grilled asparagus spears with the lemon aioli sauce for a flavorful and nutrient-packed lunch.

Dinner - Turkey and Vegetable Stir-Fry:

Ingredients:

- 1 pound ground turkey

- 1 tablespoon vegetable oil

- 1 cup broccoli florets

- 1 cup sliced bell peppers (red, green, or yellow)

- 1 cup sliced carrots

- 1 cup snap peas

- 2 tablespoons low-sodium soy sauce

- 1 tablespoon oyster sauce (optional, omit for a gluten-free version)

- 1 teaspoon grated ginger

- 2 cloves garlic, minced

- 1/4 cup chopped green onions (scallions)

- Sesame seeds for garnish

Preparation:

1. In a large skillet or wok, heat vegetable oil over medium-high heat.

2. Add ground turkey to the skillet and cook until browned and fully cooked. Remove the cooked turkey from the skillet and set aside.

3. In the same skillet, add more oil if needed, then add grated ginger and minced garlic. Sauté for about 30 seconds until fragrant.

4. Add sliced bell peppers, sliced carrots, and snap peas to the skillet. Stir-fry the vegetables for about 3-4 minutes until they become slightly tender but still crisp.

5. Return the cooked ground turkey to the skillet with the vegetables.

6. In a small bowl, mix low-sodium soy sauce and oyster sauce (if using) to create the stir-fry sauce.

7. Pour the stir-fry sauce over the turkey and vegetables in the skillet. Toss everything together to coat the ingredients with the sauce.

8. Stir-fry for another minute or two until the sauce has evenly coated the turkey and vegetables and everything is heated through.

9. Sprinkle chopped green onions and sesame seeds over the stir-fry for added flavor and garnish.

10. Serve this flavorful and protein-packed turkey and vegetable stir-fry over cooked brown rice or cauliflower rice for a nutritious dinner.

Day 9:

Breakfast - Blueberry and
Spinach Smoothie:

Ingredients:

- 1 cup fresh or frozen blueberries

- 1 cup fresh baby spinach leaves

- 1 ripe banana

- 1 cup unsweetened almond milk (or any
milk of choice)

- 1 tablespoon almond butter or peanut
butter (optional, for added creaminess)

- 1 teaspoon honey or maple syrup
(optional, for added sweetness)

- Ice cubes (optional, for a colder smoothie)

Preparation:

1. In a blender, combine blueberries, baby
spinach leaves, ripe banana, unsweetened

almond milk, almond butter or peanut butter (if using), and honey or maple syrup (if desired).

2. Blend until all the ingredients are smooth and well combined.

3. Add ice cubes if you prefer a colder and thicker smoothie and blend again until smooth.

4. Pour the blueberry and spinach smoothie into a glass and enjoy this nutrient-packed and refreshing breakfast.

Lunch - Quinoa Salad with Roasted Vegetables:

Ingredients:

- 1 cup cooked quinoa (follow package instructions)
- 1 cup diced butternut squash
- 1 cup diced sweet potatoes
- 1 cup sliced Brussels sprouts
- 1 tablespoon olive oil
- Salt and pepper to taste
- 1/4 cup dried cranberries
- 1/4 cup chopped pecans or walnuts
- 2 tablespoons balsamic vinegar
- 1 tablespoon honey (optional, for added sweetness)
- 1 teaspoon Dijon mustard
- Fresh parsley for garnish

Preparation:

1. Preheat the oven to 400°F (200°C).

2. Toss diced butternut squash, diced sweet potatoes, and sliced Brussels sprouts with olive oil, salt, and pepper on a baking sheet.

3. Roast the vegetables in the preheated oven for about 20-25 minutes or until they are tender and slightly caramelized.

4. In a large bowl, combine cooked quinoa, roasted vegetables, dried cranberries, and chopped pecans or walnuts.

5. In a separate bowl, whisk together balsamic vinegar, honey (if using), and Dijon mustard to create the dressing.

6. Pour the dressing over the quinoa and roasted vegetable mixture, tossing everything together to coat.

7. Garnish with fresh parsley before serving this colorful and nutritious quinoa salad for lunch.

Dinner - Shrimp and Zucchini Noodles Stir-Fry:

Ingredients:

- 1 pound medium-sized shrimp, peeled and deveined

- 3 medium zucchinis, spiralized or cut into thin noodles

- 1 cup sliced bell peppers (red, green, or yellow)

- 1 cup sliced mushrooms

- 2 cloves garlic, minced

- 1 tablespoon grated ginger

- 2 tablespoons low-sodium soy sauce

- 1 tablespoon oyster sauce (optional, omit for a gluten-free version)

- 1 tablespoon sesame oil

- 1 tablespoon vegetable oil

- 1/4 cup chopped green onions (scallions)

- Sesame seeds for garnish

Preparation:

1. In a large skillet or wok, heat vegetable oil over medium-high heat.

2. Add minced garlic and grated ginger to the skillet. Sauté for about 30 seconds until fragrant.

3. Add sliced bell peppers and sliced mushrooms to the skillet. Stir-fry the vegetables for about 3-4 minutes until they become slightly tender but still crisp.

4. Push the vegetables to one side of the skillet and add sesame oil to the empty space.

5. Add the shrimp to the skillet and cook for about 2-3 minutes on each side until they are pink and fully cooked.

6. In a small bowl, mix low-sodium soy sauce and oyster sauce (if using) to create the stir-fry sauce.

7. Pour the stir-fry sauce over the shrimp and vegetables in the skillet. Toss

everything together to coat the ingredients with the sauce.

8. Add zucchini noodles to the skillet and stir-fry for another minute or two until the noodles are slightly softened but still retain some crunch.

9. Sprinkle chopped green onions and sesame seeds over the stir-fry for added flavor and garnish.

10. Serve this delicious and low-carb shrimp and zucchini noodles stir-fry for a light and flavorful dinner.

Day 10:

Breakfast - Banana Nut Oatmeal:

Ingredients:

- 1 cup old-fashioned oats

- 2 cups water or milk (regular or plant-based)

- 1 ripe banana, mashed

- 1/4 cup chopped nuts (walnuts, almonds, or pecans)

- 1 tablespoon honey or maple syrup (optional, for added sweetness)

- Pinch of ground cinnamon

- Pinch of salt

Preparation:

1. In a saucepan, combine oats and water or milk.

2. Bring the mixture to a boil, then reduce the heat to low and simmer for about 5-7 minutes until the oats are tender and have absorbed most of the liquid.

3. Stir in mashed banana, chopped nuts, honey or maple syrup (if desired), ground cinnamon, and a pinch of salt.

4. Continue to cook for another minute or two until the banana is fully incorporated and the oatmeal reaches your desired consistency.

5. Serve the warm and comforting banana nut oatmeal for a satisfying breakfast.

Lunch - Spinach and Feta Stuffed Chicken Breast:

Ingredients:

- 2 boneless, skinless chicken breasts

- 1 cup fresh baby spinach leaves

- 1/4 cup crumbled feta cheese

- 1 tablespoon olive oil

- 1 teaspoon dried oregano

- 1/2 teaspoon garlic powder

- Salt and pepper to taste

Preparation:

1. Preheat the oven to 375°F (190°C). Grease a baking dish.

2. Lay the chicken breasts on a cutting board and make a horizontal slit in the thickest part of each breast to create a pocket for stuffing.

3. Stuff each chicken breast with fresh baby spinach leaves and crumbled feta cheese, evenly distributing the filling.

4. Secure the pocket with toothpicks to keep the stuffing in place.

5. Drizzle olive oil over the chicken breasts and sprinkle with dried oregano, garlic powder, salt, and pepper.

6. Heat an oven-safe skillet over medium-high heat and sear the chicken

breasts for about 2-3 minutes on each side until they develop a golden crust.

7. Transfer the skillet with the seared chicken breasts to the preheated oven and bake for about 15-20 minutes or until the chicken is cooked through and reaches an internal temperature of 165°F (74°C).

8. Remove the toothpicks before serving the flavorful and tender spinach and feta stuffed chicken breasts for lunch.

Dinner - Grilled Vegetable and Quinoa Bowl:

Ingredients:

- 1 cup cooked quinoa (follow package instructions)

- 1 cup sliced zucchini

- 1 cup sliced eggplant

- 1 cup sliced red onions

- 1 cup cherry tomatoes

- 1 tablespoon olive oil

- Salt and pepper to taste

- 2 tablespoons balsamic vinegar

- 1/4 cup crumbled goat cheese

- Fresh basil leaves for garnish

Preparation:

1. Preheat the grill or grill pan over medium-high heat.

2. Toss sliced zucchini, sliced eggplant, sliced red onions, and cherry tomatoes with olive oil, salt, and pepper in a bowl until they are evenly coated.

3. Grill the vegetables for about 5-7 minutes, turning occasionally, until they are lightly charred and tender.

4. In a large bowl, combine cooked quinoa and grilled vegetables.

5. Drizzle balsamic vinegar over the quinoa and vegetables and toss everything together to combine.

6. Sprinkle crumbled goat cheese over the bowl and garnish with fresh basil leaves before serving this colorful and nutritious grilled vegetable and quinoa bowl for dinner.

Day 11:

Breakfast - Greek Yogurt Parfait with Berries and Granola:

Ingredients:

- 1 cup plain Greek yogurt (low-fat or non-fat)

- 1/2 cup mixed fresh berries (blueberries, strawberries, raspberries)

- 1/4 cup granola (low-sugar or homemade)

- 1 tablespoon honey or maple syrup (optional, for added sweetness)

Preparation:

1. In a serving glass or bowl, layer plain Greek yogurt, mixed fresh berries, and granola.

2. Drizzle honey or maple syrup (if desired) over the parfait for added sweetness.

3. Serve this protein-rich and satisfying Greek yogurt parfait as a nutritious breakfast.

Lunch - Lentil and Kale Salad with Lemon Dressing:

Ingredients:

- 1 cup cooked green lentils (follow package instructions)
- 2 cups chopped kale leaves
- 1/4 cup diced cucumber
- 1/4 cup diced red bell pepper
- 1/4 cup diced red onion
- 1/4 cup crumbled feta cheese
- 1/4 cup chopped walnuts or almonds
- 2 tablespoons fresh lemon juice
- 2 tablespoons olive oil
- 1 teaspoon Dijon mustard
- 1 teaspoon honey or maple syrup (optional, for added sweetness)
- Salt and pepper to taste

Preparation:

1. In a large bowl, combine cooked green lentils, chopped kale leaves, diced cucumber, diced red bell pepper, diced red onion, crumbled feta cheese, and chopped walnuts or almonds.

2. In a separate small bowl, whisk together fresh lemon juice, olive oil, Dijon mustard, honey or maple syrup (if desired), salt, and pepper to create the lemon dressing.

3. Pour the lemon dressing over the lentil and kale salad and toss everything together to coat.

4. Serve this refreshing and nutrient-packed lentil and kale salad for a light and delicious lunch.

Dinner – Baked Cod with Lemon and Herbs:

Ingredients:

- 2 cod fillets (about 6 ounces each)

- 1 tablespoon olive oil

- Zest and juice of 1 lemon

- 2 cloves garlic, minced

- 1 tablespoon chopped fresh parsley

- 1 teaspoon dried dill

- Salt and pepper to taste

- Lemon slices for garnish

Preparation:

1. Preheat the oven to 375°F (190°C). Grease a baking dish or line it with parchment paper.

2. In a small bowl, mix together olive oil, lemon zest, lemon juice, minced garlic,

chopped fresh parsley, dried dill, salt, and pepper to create the marinade.

3. Place the cod fillets in the baking dish.

4. Pour the marinade over the cod fillets, making sure they are evenly coated.

5. Arrange lemon slices on top of the cod fillets for extra flavor.

6. Cover the baking dish with foil and bake in the preheated oven for about 15-20 minutes or until the cod is cooked through and easily flakes with a fork.

7. Remove the foil and bake for an additional 5 minutes to lightly brown the top.

8. Serve the baked cod with lemon and herbs with a side of steamed vegetables or a quinoa salad for a flavorful and wholesome dinner.

Day 12:

Breakfast - Mixed Berry

Smoothie Bowl:

Ingredients:

- 1 cup mixed frozen berries (blueberries, strawberries, raspberries)
- 1 ripe banana
- 1/2 cup plain Greek yogurt (low-fat or non-fat)
- 1/4 cup unsweetened almond milk (or any milk of choice)
- 1 tablespoon honey or maple syrup (optional, for added sweetness)
- Toppings: Fresh berries, sliced bananas, granola, chia seeds

Preparation:

1. In a blender, combine mixed frozen berries, ripe banana, plain Greek yogurt, unsweetened almond milk, and honey or maple syrup (if desired).

2. Blend until the mixture is smooth and creamy.

3. Pour the mixed berry smoothie into a bowl.

4. Top the smoothie bowl with fresh berries, sliced bananas, granola, and chia seeds for added texture and flavor.

5. Enjoy this vibrant and nutrient-rich mixed berry smoothie bowl for a nourishing breakfast.

Lunch - Quinoa and Avocado Salad:

Ingredients:

- 1 cup cooked quinoa (follow package instructions)
- 1 ripe avocado, diced
- 1 cup cherry tomatoes, halved
- 1/4 cup diced red onion
- 1/4 cup chopped fresh cilantro
- 2 tablespoons lime juice
- 2 tablespoons olive oil
- Salt and pepper to taste

Preparation:

1. In a large bowl, combine cooked quinoa, diced avocado, halved cherry tomatoes, diced red onion, and chopped fresh cilantro.

2. In a separate small bowl, whisk together lime juice, olive oil, salt and pepper to create the dressing.

3. Pour the dressing over the quinoa and avocado salad and toss everything together to coat.

4. Serve this light and refreshing quinoa and avocado salad for a satisfying and nutrient-packed lunch.

Dinner - Baked Chicken with Roasted Vegetables:

Ingredients:

- 2 bone-in, skin-on chicken breasts

- 1 tablespoon olive oil

- 1 teaspoon dried rosemary

- 1 teaspoon dried thyme

- 1/2 teaspoon garlic powder

- Salt and pepper to taste

- 1 cup cherry tomatoes

- 1 cup chopped broccoli florets

- 1 cup chopped cauliflower florets

- 1 tablespoon balsamic vinegar

- Fresh parsley for garnish

Preparation:

1. Preheat the oven to 400°F (200°C). Grease a baking dish.

2. Place the bone-in, skin-on chicken breasts in the baking dish.

3. Drizzle olive oil over the chicken breasts and rub them with dried rosemary, dried thyme, garlic powder, salt, and pepper, making sure they are well seasoned.

4. In a separate bowl, toss cherry tomatoes, chopped broccoli florets, and chopped cauliflower florets with olive oil, salt, and pepper.

5. Arrange the seasoned chicken breasts and the seasoned vegetables in the same baking dish.

6. Roast in the preheated oven for about 30-35 minutes or until the chicken is fully cooked and the vegetables are tender.

7. Drizzle balsamic vinegar over the roasted vegetables for added flavor.

8. Garnish with fresh parsley before serving this wholesome and tasty baked chicken with roasted vegetables for dinner.

Day 13:

Breakfast - Coconut and Mango Chia Pudding:

Ingredients:

- 1/4 cup chia seeds

- 1 cup coconut milk (canned or carton)

- 1 tablespoon honey or maple syrup (optional, for added sweetness)

- 1/2 cup diced ripe mango

- 2 tablespoons shredded coconut (unsweetened)

Preparation:

1. In a bowl, mix chia seeds with coconut milk.

2. Add honey or maple syrup (if desired) and stir well.

3. Cover the bowl and refrigerate for at least 4 hours or overnight to allow the chia seeds to absorb the liquid and form a pudding-like consistency.

4. Before serving, give the chia seed pudding a good stir.

5. Top the chia seed pudding with diced ripe mango and shredded coconut for a tropical and nutritious breakfast.

Lunch - Quinoa and Black Bean Stuffed Bell Peppers:

Ingredients:

- 2 large bell peppers (any color), halved and seeds removed
- 1 cup cooked quinoa (follow package instructions)
- 1 can (15 ounces) black beans, drained and rinsed
- 1 cup diced tomatoes
- 1 cup corn kernels (fresh, frozen, or canned)
- 1 teaspoon ground cumin
- 1/2 teaspoon chili powder
- Salt and pepper to taste
- 1/4 cup shredded cheddar cheese (reduced-fat if preferred)
- Fresh cilantro for garnish

Preparation:

1. Preheat the oven to 375°F (190°C). Grease a baking dish.

2. In a bowl, mix cooked quinoa, black beans, diced tomatoes, corn kernels, ground cumin, chili powder, salt, and pepper until well combined.

3. Stuff the halved bell peppers with the quinoa and black bean mixture, pressing down gently to fill each pepper evenly.

4. Sprinkle shredded cheddar cheese over the stuffed bell peppers for added flavor.

5. Place the stuffed bell peppers in the prepared baking dish and cover with foil.

6. Bake in the preheated oven for about 25-30 minutes or until the peppers are tender and the filling is heated through.

7. Remove the foil and bake for an additional 5 minutes to lightly melt the cheese.

8. Garnish with fresh cilantro before serving these delicious and protein-rich quinoa and black bean stuffed bell peppers for lunch.

Dinner - Vegetable and Tofu Stir-Fry:

Ingredients:

- 1 block firm tofu, drained and cubed

- 2 tablespoons low-sodium soy sauce

- 1 tablespoon cornstarch

- 1 tablespoon vegetable oil

- 1 cup sliced bell peppers (any color)

- 1 cup sliced mushrooms

- 1 cup broccoli florets

- 1 cup snap peas

- 2 cloves garlic, minced

- 1 tablespoon grated ginger

- 2 tablespoons hoisin sauce

- 1 tablespoon sesame oil

- 2 tablespoons chopped green onions (scallions)

- Sesame seeds for garnish

Preparation:

1. In a bowl, toss cubed tofu with low-sodium soy sauce and cornstarch until the tofu is evenly coated.

2. In a large skillet or wok, heat vegetable oil over medium-high heat.

3. Add the coated tofu to the skillet and cook for about 2-3 minutes on each side until the tofu becomes crispy and golden.

4. Remove the cooked tofu from the skillet and set aside.

5. In the same skillet, add more oil if needed, then add sliced bell peppers, sliced mushrooms, broccoli florets, and snap peas. Stir-fry the vegetables for about 3-4 minutes until they become slightly tender but still crisp.

6. Push the vegetables to one side of the skillet and add sesame oil to the empty space.

7. Add minced garlic and grated ginger to the skillet. Sauté for about 30 seconds until fragrant.

8. Return the cooked tofu to the skillet with the vegetables.

9. In a small bowl, mix hoisin sauce and a splash of water to create the stir-fry sauce.

10. Pour the stir-fry sauce over the tofu and vegetables in the skillet. Toss everything together to coat the ingredients with the sauce.

11. Stir-fry for another minute or two until the sauce has evenly coated the tofu and vegetables and everything is heated through.

12. Sprinkle chopped green onions and sesame seeds over the stir-fry for added flavor and garnish.

13. Serve this flavorful and plant-based vegetable and tofu stir-fry over cooked brown rice or quinoa for a satisfying dinner.

Day 14:

Breakfast - Chocolate Banana Protein Smoothie:

Ingredients:

- 1 ripe banana

- 1 cup unsweetened almond milk (or any milk of choice)

- 1 scoop chocolate protein powder (low-sugar or plant-based)

- 1 tablespoon almond butter or peanut butter

- 1 tablespoon cocoa powder (unsweetened)

- 1 teaspoon honey or maple syrup (optional, for added sweetness)

- Ice cubes (optional, for a colder smoothie)

Preparation:

1. In a blender, combine ripe banana, unsweetened almond milk, chocolate protein powder, almond butter or peanut butter, cocoa powder, and honey or maple syrup (if desired).

2. Blend until the mixture is smooth and creamy.

3. Add ice cubes if you prefer a colder and thicker smoothie and blend again until smooth.

4. Pour the chocolate banana protein smoothie into a glass and enjoy this delicious and protein-packed breakfast.

Lunch - Mediterranean Quinoa Salad:

Ingredients:

- 1 cup cooked quinoa (follow package instructions)
- 1 cup diced cucumber
- 1 cup cherry tomatoes, halved
- 1/4 cup crumbled feta cheese
- 1/4 cup sliced Kalamata olives
- 1/4 cup chopped fresh parsley
- 2 tablespoons lemon juice
- 2 tablespoons olive oil
- 1 teaspoon dried oregano
- Salt and pepper to taste

Preparation:

1. In a large bowl, combine cooked quinoa, diced cucumber, halved cherry tomatoes, crumbled feta cheese, sliced Kalamata olives, and chopped fresh parsley.

2. In a separate small bowl, whisk together lemon juice, olive oil, dried oregano, salt, and pepper to create the dressing.

3. Pour the dressing over the quinoa salad and toss everything together to coat.

4. Serve this flavorful and colorful Mediterranean quinoa salad for a light and satisfying lunch.

Dinner – Salmon with Lemon Dill Sauce and Steamed Vegetables:

Ingredients:

- 2 salmon fillets (about 6 ounces each)

- 1 tablespoon olive oil

- Zest and juice of 1 lemon

- 1 teaspoon dried dill

- 1/2 teaspoon garlic powder

- Salt and pepper to taste

For Lemon Dill Sauce:

- 1/4 cup plain Greek yogurt (low-fat or non-fat)

- Zest and juice of 1 lemon

- 1 tablespoon chopped fresh dill

- Salt and pepper to taste

For Steamed Vegetables:

- 1 cup broccoli florets

- 1 cup cauliflower florets

- 1 cup carrot slices

- 1 tablespoon olive oil

- Salt and pepper to taste

Preparation:

1. Preheat the oven to 375°F (190°C). Grease a baking dish or line it with parchment paper.

2. Place the salmon fillets in the baking dish.

3. Drizzle olive oil over the salmon fillets and rub them with lemon zest, lemon juice, dried dill, garlic powder, salt, and pepper, making sure they are well seasoned.

4. Cover the baking dish with foil and bake in the preheated oven for about 15-20 minutes or until the salmon is cooked through and easily flakes with a fork.

5. While the salmon is baking, prepare the lemon dill sauce. In a small bowl, whisk together plain Greek yogurt, lemon zest, lemon juice, chopped fresh dill, salt, and pepper to create the sauce. Set aside.

6. For the steamed vegetables, place a steamer basket in a pot with a few inches of water. Bring the water to a boil, then add broccoli florets, cauliflower florets, and carrot slices to the steamer basket.

7. Cover the pot with a lid and steam the vegetables for about 5-7 minutes until they are tender but still retain some crunch.

8. Drizzle olive oil over the steamed vegetables and season with salt and pepper to taste.

9. Remove the foil from the baked salmon and continue to bake for an additional 5 minutes to lightly brown the top.

10. Serve the baked salmon with lemon dill sauce and steamed vegetables for a delicious and nutritious dinner.

Day 15:

Breakfast - Apple Cinnamon Overnight Oats:

Ingredients:

- 1/2 cup rolled oats

- 1/2 cup unsweetened almond milk (or any milk of choice)

- 1/2 cup unsweetened applesauce

- 1 tablespoon maple syrup or honey

- 1/2 teaspoon ground cinnamon

- 1/4 teaspoon vanilla extract

- 1/4 cup diced apple

- 1 tablespoon chopped nuts (walnuts or almonds)

Preparation:

1. In a jar or container with a lid, combine rolled oats, unsweetened almond milk,

unsweetened applesauce, maple syrup or honey, ground cinnamon, and vanilla extract.

2. Stir well to ensure all the ingredients are well mixed.

3. Add diced apple and chopped nuts on top.

4. Cover the jar or container and refrigerate overnight to allow the oats to soften and absorb the flavors.

5. In the morning, give the overnight oats a good stir and enjoy this delicious and fuss-free breakfast.

Lunch - Caprese Salad with Balsamic Glaze:

Ingredients:

- 1 cup cherry tomatoes, halved

- 1 cup fresh mozzarella balls, halved

- 1/4 cup fresh basil leaves, torn

- 2 tablespoons balsamic glaze

- 1 tablespoon extra-virgin olive oil

- Salt and pepper to taste

Preparation:

1. In a bowl, combine halved cherry tomatoes and fresh mozzarella balls.

2. Toss torn fresh basil leaves with the tomato and mozzarella mixture.

3. Drizzle balsamic glaze and extra-virgin olive oil over the salad.

4. Season with salt and pepper to taste.

5. Toss everything together to combine.

6. Serve this classic and flavorful Caprese salad for a light and refreshing lunch.

Dinner - Eggplant Parmesan with Marinara Sauce:

Ingredients:

- 2 large eggplants, sliced into rounds
- 2 cups marinara sauce (store-bought or homemade)
- 1 cup shredded mozzarella cheese
- 1/2 cup grated Parmesan cheese
- 1/4 cup chopped fresh basil
- 1 tablespoon olive oil
- Salt and pepper to taste

Preparation:

1. Preheat the oven to 375°F (190°C). Grease a baking dish.

2. Lay the eggplant slices on a baking sheet and brush both sides with olive oil. Season with salt and pepper.

3. Bake the eggplant slices in the preheated oven for about 10-12 minutes until they are slightly tender.

4. In the greased baking dish, spread a layer of marinara sauce on the bottom.

5. Arrange a layer of baked eggplant slices over the marinara sauce.

6. Sprinkle shredded mozzarella cheese and grated Parmesan cheese over the eggplant slices.

7. Repeat the layers, ending with a layer of marinara sauce and cheeses on top.

8. Bake in the preheated oven for about 20-25 minutes or until the cheese is melted and bubbly, and the eggplant is fully cooked.

9. Remove the eggplant Parmesan from the oven and let it cool for a few minutes.

10. Sprinkle chopped fresh basil over the top before serving this comforting and cheesy eggplant Parmesan for dinner.

Day 16:

Breakfast - Veggie Omelette:

Ingredients:

- 3 large eggs

- 1/4 cup diced bell peppers (any color)

- 1/4 cup diced onions

- 1/4 cup diced tomatoes

- 1/4 cup sliced mushrooms

- 1/4 cup shredded cheddar cheese

- 1 tablespoon chopped fresh parsley

- Salt and pepper to taste

- 1 tablespoon olive oil

Preparation:

1. In a bowl, beat the eggs and season with salt and pepper.

2. In a non-stick skillet, heat olive oil over medium-high heat.

3. Add diced bell peppers, onions, tomatoes, and sliced mushrooms to the skillet. Sauté for about 3-4 minutes until the vegetables become slightly tender.

4. Pour the beaten eggs over the sautéed vegetables in the skillet.

5. Sprinkle shredded cheddar cheese and chopped fresh parsley over the eggs.

6. Cook the omelette for a few minutes until the edges are set and the cheese starts to melt.

7. Carefully flip one side of the omelette over the other to fold it in half.

8. Cook for another minute or two until the eggs are fully cooked and the cheese is melted.

9. Slide the veggie omelette onto a plate and serve it as a wholesome and protein-rich breakfast.

Lunch - Chicken and Avocado Wrap:

Ingredients:

- 1 grilled chicken breast, sliced

- 1 large whole wheat tortilla or wrap

- 1/2 avocado, sliced

- 1/4 cup sliced cucumbers

- 1/4 cup shredded lettuce

- 1 tablespoon Greek yogurt or light mayo (optional, for added creaminess)

- 1 teaspoon lime juice

- Salt and pepper to taste

Preparation:

1. Lay the whole wheat tortilla or wrap on a clean surface.

2. In the center of the tortilla, arrange the sliced grilled chicken breast, sliced

avocado, sliced cucumbers, and shredded lettuce.

3. In a small bowl, mix Greek yogurt or light mayo (if using) with lime juice, salt, and pepper to create the dressing.

4. Drizzle the dressing over the chicken and avocado filling.

5. Fold in the sides of the tortilla and roll it up tightly to form a wrap.

6. Slice the chicken and avocado wrap in half and serve it for a satisfying and portable lunch.

Dinner - Stir-Fried Tofu with Broccoli and Cashews:

Ingredients:

- 1 block firm tofu, cubed

- 1 tablespoon cornstarch

- 1/4 cup low-sodium soy sauce

- 2 tablespoons hoisin sauce

- 1 tablespoon rice vinegar

- 1 tablespoon brown sugar or honey

- 1 tablespoon vegetable oil

- 2 cups broccoli florets

- 1/2 cup roasted cashews

- 2 cloves garlic, minced

- 1 tablespoon grated ginger

- 1/4 cup chopped green onions (scallions)

- Sesame seeds for garnish

Preparation:

1. In a bowl, toss cubed tofu with cornstarch until the tofu is evenly coated.

2. In a separate small bowl, mix low-sodium soy sauce, hoisin sauce, rice vinegar, and brown sugar or honey to create the stir-fry sauce.

3. In a large skillet or wok, heat vegetable oil over medium-high heat.

4. Add the coated tofu to the skillet and cook for about 2-3 minutes on each side until the tofu becomes crispy and golden.

5. Remove the cooked tofu from the skillet and set aside.

6. In the same skillet, add more oil if needed, then add minced garlic and grated ginger. Sauté for about 30 seconds until fragrant.

7. Add broccoli florets to the skillet. Stir-fry the broccoli for about 3-4 minutes until it becomes slightly tender but still crisp.

8. Return the cooked tofu to the skillet with the broccoli.

9. Pour the stir-fry sauce over the tofu and broccoli in the skillet. Toss everything together to coat the ingredients with the sauce.

10. Stir-fry for another minute or two until the sauce has evenly coated the tofu and broccoli and everything is heated through.

11. Add roasted cashews to the skillet and toss everything together.

12. Sprinkle chopped green onions and sesame seeds over the stir-fry for added flavor and garnish.

13. Serve this flavorful and plant-based stir-fried tofu with broccoli and cashews over cooked brown rice or quinoa for a delicious and nutritious dinner.

Day 17

Breakfast - Peanut Butter and Banana Toast:

Ingredients:

- 2 slices whole grain bread
- 2 tablespoons natural peanut butter
- 1 ripe banana, sliced
- 1 tablespoon honey (optional, for added sweetness)

Preparation:

1. Toast the whole grain bread slices until they are golden and crispy.

2. Spread natural peanut butter evenly over each toast slice.

3. Arrange sliced banana over the peanut butter layer.

4. Drizzle honey over the top (if desired) for added sweetness.

5. Enjoy this simple and satisfying peanut butter and banana toast for breakfast.

Lunch - Lentil and Vegetable Soup:

Ingredients:

- 1 cup cooked green lentils (follow package instructions)
- 1 tablespoon olive oil
- 1 cup diced onions
- 1 cup diced carrots
- 1 cup diced celery
- 2 cloves garlic, minced
- 1 teaspoon ground cumin
- 1/2 teaspoon paprika

- 1/4 teaspoon cayenne pepper (optional, for spiciness)
- 4 cups low-sodium vegetable broth
- 1 can (14 ounces) diced tomatoes
- Salt and pepper to taste
- Fresh parsley for garnish

Preparation:

1. In a large pot, heat olive oil over medium-high heat.

2. Add diced onions, diced carrots, and diced celery to the pot. Sauté for about 3-4 minutes until the vegetables become slightly tender.

3. Add minced garlic, ground cumin, paprika, and cayenne pepper (if using) to the pot. Sauté for another 30 seconds until fragrant.

4. Pour low-sodium vegetable broth into the pot.

5. Add cooked green lentils and diced tomatoes (with their juices) to the pot.

6. Bring the soup to a boil, then reduce the heat to low and let it simmer for about 15-20 minutes to allow the flavors to meld together.

7. Season the soup with salt and pepper to taste.

8. Ladle the lentil and vegetable soup into bowls and garnish with fresh parsley before serving this hearty and nutritious lunch.

Dinner - Shrimp and Asparagus Stir-Fry:

Ingredients:

- 1 pound medium-sized shrimp, peeled and deveined
- 1 bunch asparagus, trimmed and cut into pieces

- 1 cup sliced bell peppers (any color)

- 1 cup sliced carrots

- 2 tablespoons low-sodium soy sauce

- 1 tablespoon oyster sauce (optional, omit for a gluten-free version)

- 1 tablespoon sesame oil

- 1 tablespoon vegetable oil

- 2 cloves garlic, minced

- 1 tablespoon grated ginger

- 1/4 cup chopped green onions (scallions)

- Sesame seeds for garnish

Preparation:

1. In a bowl, mix shrimp with low-sodium soy sauce and set aside to marinate for a few minutes.

2. In a large skillet or wok, heat vegetable oil and sesame oil over medium-high heat.

3. Add minced garlic and grated ginger to the skillet. Sauté for about 30 seconds until fragrant.

4. Add sliced bell peppers and sliced carrots to the skillet. Stir-fry the vegetables for about 3-4 minutes until they become slightly tender but still crisp.

5. Push the vegetables to one side of the skillet and add the marinated shrimp to the empty space.

6. Stir-fry the shrimp for about 2-3 minutes until they turn pink and are fully cooked.

7. Combine the cooked shrimp with the stir-fried vegetables in the skillet.

8. Add asparagus pieces to the skillet and continue to stir-fry for another 2 minutes until the asparagus becomes tender but still retains some crunch.

9. If using oyster sauce, drizzle it over the stir-fried shrimp and vegetables and toss everything together to coat. If omitting oyster sauce, you can add a splash of extra low-sodium soy sauce for extra flavor.

10. Stir-fry for another minute to evenly coat the ingredients with the sauce and to heat everything through.

11. Sprinkle chopped green onions and sesame seeds over the stir-fry for added flavor and garnish.

12. Serve this quick and flavorful shrimp and asparagus stir-fry over cooked brown rice or quinoa for a satisfying dinner.

Day 18

Breakfast - Blueberry Almond Overnight Oats:

Ingredients:

- 1/2 cup rolled oats

- 1/2 cup unsweetened almond milk (or any milk of choice)

- 1/4 cup fresh blueberries

- 2 tablespoons sliced almonds

- 1 tablespoon honey or maple syrup (optional, for added sweetness)

Preparation:

1. In a jar or container with a lid, combine rolled oats and unsweetened almond milk.

2. Add fresh blueberries and sliced almonds on top.

3. Drizzle honey or maple syrup (if desired) over the oats.

4. Cover the jar or container and refrigerate overnight to allow the oats to soften and absorb the flavors.

5. In the morning, give the blueberry almond overnight oats a good stir and enjoy this nutritious and delicious breakfast.

Lunch - Quinoa and Chickpea Salad:

Ingredients:

- 1 cup cooked quinoa (follow package instructions)

- 1 can (15 ounces) chickpeas, drained and rinsed

- 1/2 cup diced cucumbers

- 1/2 cup diced red bell pepper

- 1/4 cup chopped fresh parsley

- 2 tablespoons lemon juice

- 2 tablespoons olive oil

- 1 teaspoon ground cumin

- Salt and pepper to taste

Preparation:

1. In a large bowl, combine cooked quinoa, chickpeas, diced cucumbers, diced red bell pepper, and chopped fresh parsley.

2. In a separate small bowl, whisk together lemon juice, olive oil, ground cumin, salt, and pepper to create the dressing.

3. Pour the dressing over the quinoa and chickpea salad and toss everything together to coat.

4. Serve this protein-rich and refreshing quinoa and chickpea salad for a light and satisfying lunch.

Dinner - Baked Turkey Meatballs with Zucchini Noodles:

Ingredients:

For Turkey Meatballs:

- 1 pound ground turkey

- 1/4 cup breadcrumbs (whole wheat or gluten-free)

- 1/4 cup grated Parmesan cheese

- 1/4 cup chopped fresh parsley

- 1 egg

- 2 cloves garlic, minced

- 1 teaspoon dried oregano

- 1 teaspoon dried basil

- Salt and pepper to taste

For Zucchini Noodles:

- 3 medium zucchini, spiralized or thinly sliced

- 1 tablespoon olive oil

- 2 cloves garlic, minced

- Salt and pepper to taste

For Marinara Sauce:

- 2 cups marinara sauce (store-bought or homemade)

- 1/4 cup chopped fresh basil

- 1/4 cup grated Parmesan cheese

Preparation:

1. Preheat the oven to 400°F (200°C). Line a baking sheet with parchment paper.

2. In a bowl, mix ground turkey, breadcrumbs, grated Parmesan cheese, chopped fresh parsley, egg, minced garlic,

dried oregano, dried basil, salt, and pepper until well combined.

3. Shape the turkey mixture into meatballs and place them on the prepared baking sheet.

4. Bake the turkey meatballs in the preheated oven for about 15-20 minutes or until they are cooked through and lightly browned.

5. While the meatballs are baking, prepare the zucchini noodles. In a large skillet, heat olive oil over medium heat.

6. Add minced garlic to the skillet and sauté for about 30 seconds until fragrant.

7. Add spiralized or thinly sliced zucchini to the skillet. Stir-fry for about 3-4 minutes until the zucchini becomes slightly tender but still retains some crunch.

8. Season the zucchini noodles with salt and pepper to taste.

9. In a separate saucepan, heat marinara sauce over medium heat until it is heated through.

10. Once the turkey meatballs are cooked, add them to the marinara sauce and toss everything together to coat the meatballs with the sauce.

11. Serve the baked turkey meatballs with zucchini noodles, topped with chopped fresh basil and grated Parmesan cheese for a flavorful and nutritious dinner.

Day 19:

Breakfast - Greek Yogurt and Berry Parfait:

Ingredients:

- 1 cup plain Greek yogurt (low-fat or non-fat)
- 1/2 cup mixed fresh berries (blueberries, strawberries, raspberries)
- 1/4 cup granola (low-sugar or homemade)
- 1 tablespoon honey or maple syrup (optional, for added sweetness)

Preparation:

1. In a serving glass or bowl, layer plain Greek yogurt, mixed fresh berries, and granola.

2. Drizzle honey or maple syrup (if desired) over the parfait for added sweetness.

3. Serve this protein-rich and flavorful Greek yogurt and berry parfait as a delicious breakfast.

Lunch - Spinach and Quinoa Stuffed Bell Peppers:

Ingredients:

- 2 large bell peppers (any color), halved and seeds removed

- 1 cup cooked quinoa (follow package instructions)

- 1 cup chopped fresh spinach

- 1/2 cup diced tomatoes

- 1/4 cup diced red onion

- 1/4 cup crumbled feta cheese

- 2 tablespoons fresh lemon juice

- 2 tablespoons olive oil

- 1 teaspoon dried oregano

- Salt and pepper to taste

Preparation:

1. Preheat the oven to 375°F (190°C). Grease a baking dish.

2. In a large bowl, combine cooked quinoa, chopped fresh spinach, diced tomatoes, diced red onion, and crumbled feta cheese.

3. In a separate small bowl, whisk together fresh lemon juice, olive oil, dried oregano, salt, and pepper to create the dressing.

4. Pour the dressing over the quinoa and spinach mixture and toss everything together to coat.

5. Stuff the halved bell peppers with the quinoa and spinach mixture, pressing down gently to fill each pepper evenly.

6. Place the stuffed bell peppers in the prepared baking dish.

7. Cover the baking dish with foil and bake in the preheated oven for about 20-25 minutes or until the peppers are tender and the filling is heated through.

8. Remove the foil and bake for an additional 5 minutes to lightly brown the top.

9. Serve these nutritious and flavorful spinach and quinoa stuffed bell peppers for a satisfying lunch.

Dinner - Baked Cod with Lemon Garlic Butter:

Ingredients:

- 2 cod fillets (about 6 ounces each)

- 2 tablespoons butter, melted

- 2 cloves garlic, minced

- Zest and juice of 1 lemon

- 1 tablespoon chopped fresh parsley

- Salt and pepper to taste

For Roasted Brussels Sprouts:

- 2 cups Brussels sprouts, halved

- 1 tablespoon olive oil

- Salt and pepper to taste

Preparation:

1. Preheat the oven to 400°F (200°C). Grease a baking dish.

2. Place the cod fillets in the prepared baking dish.

3. In a small bowl, mix melted butter, minced garlic, lemon zest, lemon juice, chopped fresh parsley, salt, and pepper to create the lemon garlic butter sauce.

4. Pour the lemon garlic butter sauce over the cod fillets, coating them evenly.

5. Bake the cod in the preheated oven for about 12-15 minutes or until the fish is fully cooked and flakes easily with a fork.

6. While the cod is baking, prepare the roasted Brussels sprouts. Toss halved Brussels sprouts with olive oil, salt, and pepper on a separate baking sheet.

7. Roast the Brussels sprouts in the same oven as the cod for about 15-20 minutes until they are tender and slightly caramelized.

8. Serve the baked cod with lemon garlic butter alongside roasted Brussels sprouts for a delicious and healthy dinner.

Day 20

Breakfast - Green Smoothie Bowl:

Ingredients:

- 1 ripe banana

- 1 cup fresh spinach leaves

- 1/2 cup frozen pineapple chunks

- 1/2 cup frozen mango chunks

- 1/2 cup unsweetened almond milk (or any milk of choice)

- 1 tablespoon chia seeds

- 1 tablespoon shredded coconut (unsweetened)

- Fresh fruit and nuts for topping

Preparation:

1. In a blender, combine ripe banana, fresh spinach leaves, frozen pineapple chunks, frozen mango chunks, and unsweetened almond milk.

2. Blend until the mixture is smooth and creamy.

3. Pour the green smoothie into a bowl.

4. Sprinkle chia seeds and shredded coconut over the smoothie.

5. Top with fresh fruit and nuts of your choice, such as sliced strawberries, blueberries, and chopped almonds.

6. Enjoy this vibrant and nutrient-packed green smoothie bowl for breakfast.

Lunch - Turkey and Avocado Wrap:

Ingredients:

- 2 slices whole grain bread

- 4 slices roasted turkey breast

- 1/2 avocado, sliced

- 1/4 cup sliced cucumbers

- 1/4 cup shredded lettuce

- 1 tablespoon Greek yogurt or light mayo (optional, for added creaminess)

- 1 teaspoon lime juice

- Salt and pepper to taste

Preparation:

1. Lay the whole grain bread slices on a clean surface.

2. On each slice, layer two slices of roasted turkey breast, sliced avocado, sliced cucumbers, and shredded lettuce.

3. In a small bowl, mix Greek yogurt or light mayo (if using) with lime juice, salt, and pepper to create the dressing.

4. Drizzle the dressing over the turkey and avocado filling.

5. Fold in the sides of the bread slices and roll them up tightly to form a wrap.

6. Slice the turkey and avocado wrap in half and serve it for a satisfying and portable lunch.

Dinner - Quinoa Stuffed Bell Peppers with Black Beans:

Ingredients:

- 2 large bell peppers (any color), halved and seeds removed

- 1 cup cooked quinoa (follow package instructions)

- 1 can (15 ounces) black beans, drained and rinsed

- 1 cup diced tomatoes

- 1/2 cup diced red onion

- 1/4 cup chopped fresh cilantro

- 1 tablespoon taco seasoning

- 1/2 cup shredded cheddar cheese

- Lime wedges for serving

Preparation:

1. Preheat the oven to 375°F (190°C). Grease a baking dish.

2. In a large bowl, combine cooked quinoa, black beans, diced tomatoes, diced red onion, chopped fresh cilantro, and taco seasoning.

3. Stuff the halved bell peppers with the quinoa and black bean mixture, pressing down gently to fill each pepper evenly.

4. Place the stuffed bell peppers in the prepared baking dish.

5. Cover the baking dish with foil and bake in the preheated oven for about 20-25 minutes or until the peppers are tender and the filling is heated through.

6. Remove the foil and sprinkle shredded cheddar cheese over the stuffed bell peppers.

7. Bake for an additional 5 minutes or until the cheese is melted and bubbly.

8. Serve these delicious and protein-rich quinoa stuffed bell peppers with black

beans, garnished with fresh cilantro and lime wedges on the side.

Day 21

Breakfast - Raspberry Chia Seed Pudding:

Ingredients:

- 1/4 cup chia seeds

- 1 cup unsweetened almond milk (or any milk of choice)

- 1/2 teaspoon vanilla extract

- 1 tablespoon honey or maple syrup (optional, for added sweetness)

- 1/2 cup fresh raspberries

- 2 tablespoons sliced almonds

Preparation:

1. In a bowl, mix chia seeds with unsweetened almond milk and vanilla extract.

2. Add honey or maple syrup (if desired) and stir well.

3. Cover the bowl and refrigerate for at least 4 hours or overnight to allow the chia seeds to absorb the liquid and form a pudding-like consistency.

4. Before serving, give the chia seed pudding a good stir.

5. Top the chia seed pudding with fresh raspberries and sliced almonds for a colorful and nutritious breakfast.

Lunch - Shrimp and Avocado Salad:

Ingredients:

- 1 cup cooked shrimp, peeled and deveined

- 1 ripe avocado, diced

- 1 cup cherry tomatoes, halved

- 1/4 cup sliced red onions

- 2 tablespoons fresh lime juice

- 1 tablespoon olive oil

- 1 tablespoon chopped fresh cilantro

- Salt and pepper to taste

Preparation:

1. In a large bowl, combine cooked shrimp, diced avocado, halved cherry tomatoes, and sliced red onions.

2. In a separate small bowl, whisk together fresh lime juice, olive oil, chopped fresh

cilantro, salt, and pepper to create the dressing.

3. Pour the dressing over the shrimp and avocado salad and toss everything together to coat.

4. Serve this refreshing and protein-packed shrimp and avocado salad for a light and satisfying lunch.

Dinner - Baked Chicken and Vegetable Foil Packets:

Ingredients:

- 2 boneless, skinless chicken breasts

- 1 cup broccoli florets

- 1 cup sliced bell peppers (any color)

- 1 cup sliced zucchini

- 1 cup sliced carrots

- 2 cloves garlic, minced

- 2 tablespoons olive oil

- 2 tablespoons fresh lemon juice

- 1 teaspoon dried thyme

- Salt and pepper to taste

- Fresh parsley for garnish

Preparation:

1. Preheat the oven to 375°F (190°C).

2. Cut two large pieces of aluminum foil and place them on a baking sheet.

3. In a bowl, mix olive oil, fresh lemon juice, minced garlic, dried thyme, salt, and pepper to create the marinade.

4. Place one chicken breast in the center of each piece of aluminum foil.

5. Pour the marinade over the chicken breasts, coating them evenly.

6. Arrange broccoli florets, sliced bell peppers, sliced zucchini, and sliced carrots around each chicken breast on the foil.

7. Fold the foil over the chicken and vegetables to form a packet, sealing the edges tightly.

8. Bake the chicken and vegetable foil packets in the preheated oven for about 25-30 minutes or until the chicken is fully cooked and the vegetables are tender.

9. Carefully open the foil packets and transfer the baked chicken and vegetables to serving plates.

10. Garnish with fresh parsley before serving this delicious and wholesome dinner.

Day 22

Breakfast - Almond Butter and Banana Toast:

Ingredients:

- 2 slices whole grain bread

- 2 tablespoons natural almond butter

- 1 ripe banana, sliced

- 1 tablespoon honey (optional, for added sweetness)

Preparation:

1. Toast the whole grain bread slices until they are golden and crispy.

2. Spread natural almond butter evenly over each toast slice.

3. Arrange sliced banana over the almond butter layer.

4. Drizzle honey over the top (if desired) for added sweetness.

5. Enjoy this simple and satisfying almond butter and banana toast for breakfast.

Lunch - Lentil and Kale Soup:

Ingredients:

- 1 cup dried green lentils

- 4 cups vegetable broth

- 2 cups chopped kale

- 1 cup diced carrots

- 1 cup diced celery

- 1 cup diced onions

- 2 cloves garlic, minced

- 1 teaspoon dried thyme

- 1 bay leaf

- Salt and pepper to taste

- Fresh lemon wedges for serving

Preparation:

1. Rinse the dried green lentils under cold water and drain them.

2. In a large pot, combine lentils, vegetable broth, chopped kale, diced carrots, diced

celery, diced onions, minced garlic, dried thyme, and bay leaf.

3. Bring the soup to a boil, then reduce the heat to low and let it simmer for about 20-25 minutes or until the lentils and vegetables are tender.

4. Remove the bay leaf from the soup and season with salt and pepper to taste.

5. Ladle the lentil and kale soup into bowls and serve with fresh lemon wedges for added flavor.

Dinner - Baked Cod with Mediterranean Salsa:

Ingredients:

- 2 cod fillets (about 6 ounces each)

- 2 tablespoons olive oil

- 2 tablespoons fresh lemon juice

- 1 teaspoon dried oregano

- 1/2 teaspoon garlic powder

- Salt and pepper to taste

For Mediterranean Salsa:

- 1 cup diced tomatoes

- 1/2 cup diced cucumber

- 1/4 cup diced red onion

- 1/4 cup sliced Kalamata olives

- 2 tablespoons chopped fresh parsley

- 1 tablespoon olive oil

- 1 tablespoon red wine vinegar

- Salt and pepper to taste

Preparation:

1. Preheat the oven to 400°F (200°C). Grease a baking dish.

2. Place the cod fillets in the prepared baking dish.

3. Drizzle olive oil and fresh lemon juice over the cod fillets, coating them evenly.

4. Sprinkle dried oregano, garlic powder, salt, and pepper over the cod.

5. Bake the cod in the preheated oven for about 12-15 minutes or until the fish is fully cooked and flakes easily with a fork.

6. While the cod is baking, prepare the Mediterranean salsa. In a bowl, combine diced tomatoes, diced cucumber, diced red onion, sliced Kalamata olives, chopped fresh parsley, olive oil, red wine vinegar, salt, and pepper. Toss everything together to combine.

7. Serve the baked cod with Mediterranean salsa on top for a flavorful and light dinner.

Day 23

Breakfast - Mixed Berry Smoothie:

Ingredients:

- 1 cup mixed fresh berries (blueberries, strawberries, raspberries)
- 1 ripe banana
- 1 cup unsweetened almond milk (or any milk of choice)
- 1 tablespoon honey or maple syrup (optional, for added sweetness)
- 1 tablespoon chia seeds (optional, for added fiber and nutrients)
- Fresh mint leaves for garnish

Preparation:

1. In a blender, combine mixed fresh berries, ripe banana, and unsweetened almond milk.

2. Blend until the mixture is smooth and creamy.

3. Add honey or maple syrup (if desired) and chia seeds to the blender and blend again until well combined.

4. Pour the mixed berry smoothie into glasses.

5. Garnish with fresh mint leaves before serving this refreshing and nutrient-packed breakfast.

Lunch - Chickpea and Avocado Salad:

Ingredients:

- 1 can (15 ounces) chickpeas, drained and rinsed
- 1 ripe avocado, diced
- 1 cup cherry tomatoes, halved
- 1/4 cup diced red onion
- 2 tablespoons fresh lemon juice
- 1 tablespoon olive oil
- 1 tablespoon chopped fresh basil
- Salt and pepper to taste

Preparation:

1. In a large bowl, combine chickpeas, diced avocado, halved cherry tomatoes, and diced red onion.

2. In a separate small bowl, whisk together fresh lemon juice, olive oil, chopped fresh basil, salt, and pepper to create the dressing.

3. Pour the dressing over the chickpea and avocado salad and toss everything together to coat.

4. Serve this vibrant and protein-packed chickpea and avocado salad for a light and satisfying lunch.

Dinner - Grilled Lemon Herb Chicken with Quinoa Pilaf:

Ingredients:

For Grilled Lemon Herb Chicken:

- 2 boneless, skinless chicken breasts

- 2 tablespoons olive oil

- Zest and juice of 1 lemon

- 2 cloves garlic, minced

- 1 tablespoon chopped fresh rosemary

- 1 tablespoon chopped fresh thyme

- Salt and pepper to taste

For Quinoa Pilaf:

- 1 cup quinoa (follow package instructions)

- 1/4 cup chopped dried apricots

- 1/4 cup chopped almonds

- 2 tablespoons chopped fresh parsley

- 1 tablespoon olive oil

- Salt and pepper to taste

Preparation:

1. In a bowl, mix olive oil, lemon zest, lemon juice, minced garlic, chopped fresh rosemary, chopped fresh thyme, salt, and pepper to create the marinade for the chicken.

2. Place the chicken breasts in the marinade, coating them evenly.

3. Cover the bowl and refrigerate for at least 30 minutes to allow the chicken to marinate and absorb the flavors.

4. While the chicken is marinating, prepare the quinoa pilaf. Cook the quinoa according to the package instructions.

5. In a separate small bowl, mix chopped dried apricots, chopped almonds, chopped fresh parsley, olive oil, salt, and pepper.

6. When the quinoa is cooked, add the apricot and almond mixture to the quinoa

and toss everything together to combine. Set aside.

7. Preheat the grill or grill pan over medium-high heat.

8. Remove the chicken from the marinade and discard the excess marinade.

9. Grill the chicken breasts for about 4-5 minutes on each side, or until they are fully cooked and have grill marks.

10. Remove the grilled lemon herb chicken from the grill and let it rest for a few minutes before slicing.

11. Serve the grilled lemon herb chicken with quinoa pilaf for a flavorful and protein-packed dinner.

Day 24

Breakfast - Peanut Butter and Jelly Overnight Oats:

Ingredients:

- 1/2 cup rolled oats

- 1 cup unsweetened almond milk (or any milk of choice)

- 2 tablespoons natural peanut butter

- 2 tablespoons fruit preserves (strawberry, raspberry, or any flavor of choice)

- Fresh berries for topping

Preparation:

1. In a jar or container with a lid, combine rolled oats and unsweetened almond milk.

2. Add natural peanut butter to the oats mixture and stir well.

3. Layer fruit preserves over the oats mixture.

4. Cover the jar or container and refrigerate overnight to allow the oats to soften and absorb the flavors.

5. In the morning, give the peanut butter and jelly overnight oats a good stir.

6. Top with fresh berries before serving this delicious and nostalgic breakfast.

Lunch - Caprese Salad with Balsamic Glaze:

Ingredients:

- 1 cup cherry tomatoes, halved

- 1 cup fresh mozzarella balls, halved

- 1/2 cup fresh basil leaves

- 2 tablespoons balsamic glaze

- 2 tablespoons extra-virgin olive oil

- Salt and pepper to taste

Preparation:

1. In a large bowl, combine halved cherry tomatoes and halved fresh mozzarella balls.

2. Tear fresh basil leaves and add them to the bowl.

3. Drizzle balsamic glaze and extra-virgin olive oil over the salad.

4. Season with salt and pepper to taste.

5. Toss everything together to coat and combine.

6. Serve this simple and flavorful Caprese salad for a light and refreshing lunch.

Dinner - Veggie Stir-Fry with Tofu:

Ingredients:

- 1 block firm tofu, cubed

- 1 tablespoon cornstarch

- 2 tablespoons low-sodium soy sauce

- 1 tablespoon hoisin sauce (optional, omit for a gluten-free version)

- 1 tablespoon sesame oil

- 2 tablespoons vegetable oil

- 2 cups broccoli florets

- 1 cup sliced bell peppers (any color)

- 1 cup sliced carrots

- 1 cup snap peas

- 2 cloves garlic, minced

- 1 tablespoon grated ginger

- 1/4 cup chopped green onions (scallions)

- Sesame seeds for garnish

Preparation:

1. In a bowl, toss cubed tofu with cornstarch until the tofu is evenly coated.

2. In a separate small bowl, mix low-sodium soy sauce, hoisin sauce (if using), and sesame oil to create the stir-fry sauce.

3. In a large skillet or wok, heat vegetable oil over medium-high heat.

4. Add the coated tofu to the skillet and cook for about 2-3 minutes on each side until the tofu becomes crispy and golden.

5. Remove the cooked tofu from the skillet and set aside.

6. In the same skillet, add more oil if needed, then add minced garlic and grated ginger. Sauté for about 30 seconds until fragrant.

7. Add broccoli florets, sliced bell peppers, sliced carrots, and snap peas to the skillet.

Stir-fry the vegetables for about 3-4 minutes until they become slightly tender but still crisp.

8. Return the cooked tofu to the skillet with the vegetables.

9. Pour the stir-fry sauce over the tofu and vegetables in the skillet. Toss everything together to coat the ingredients with the sauce.

10. Stir-fry for another minute or two until the sauce has evenly coated the tofu and vegetables and everything is heated through.

11. Sprinkle chopped green onions and sesame seeds over the stir-fry for added flavor and garnish.

12. Serve this flavorful and plant-based veggie stir-fry with tofu over cooked brown rice or quinoa for a delicious and nutritious dinner.

Day 25

Ingredients:

- 1 pack frozen acai puree (unsweetened)

- 1 ripe banana

- 1/2 cup frozen mixed berries (blueberries, strawberries, raspberries)

- 1/2 cup unsweetened almond milk (or any milk of choice)

- 1 tablespoon honey or maple syrup (optional, for added sweetness)

- Fresh fruit, granola, and shredded coconut for topping

Preparation:

1. In a blender, combine frozen acai puree, ripe banana, frozen mixed berries, and unsweetened almond milk.

2. Blend until the mixture is smooth and creamy.

3. Add honey or maple syrup (if desired) and blend again until well combined.

4. Pour the acai smoothie into a bowl.

5. Top with fresh fruit, granola, and shredded coconut before serving this colorful and nutrient-packed breakfast.

Lunch - Quinoa and Black Bean Stuffed Sweet Potatoes:

Ingredients:

- 2 medium sweet potatoes

- 1 cup cooked quinoa (follow package instructions)

- 1 can (15 ounces) black beans, drained and rinsed

- 1 cup diced tomatoes

- 1/2 cup diced red onion

- 1/4 cup chopped fresh cilantro

- 1 tablespoon olive oil

- 1 tablespoon fresh lime juice

- 1 teaspoon ground cumin

- Salt and pepper to taste

- Avocado slices for topping

- Fresh cilantro for garnish

Preparation:

1. Preheat the oven to 400°F (200°C).

2. Wash the sweet potatoes and pierce them several times with a fork.

3. Place the sweet potatoes on a baking sheet and bake in the preheated oven for about 45-50 minutes or until they are tender and can be easily pierced with a fork.

4. While the sweet potatoes are baking, prepare the quinoa and black bean filling. In a large bowl, combine cooked quinoa, black beans, diced tomatoes, diced red onion, chopped fresh cilantro, olive oil, fresh lime juice, ground cumin, salt, and pepper. Toss everything together to combine.

5. Once the sweet potatoes are done baking, let them cool slightly before handling.

6. Slice the sweet potatoes open lengthwise, being careful not to cut them all the way through.

7. Gently mash the flesh of the sweet potatoes with a fork to create a pocket for the filling.

8. Spoon the quinoa and black bean filling into each sweet potato, pressing down gently to fill each potato evenly.

9. Top each stuffed sweet potato with avocado slices and fresh cilantro.

10. Serve these delicious and hearty quinoa and black bean stuffed sweet potatoes for a flavorful and nutritious lunch.

Dinner - Baked Eggplant Parmesan:

Ingredients:

- 1 large eggplant, sliced into 1/4-inch rounds

- 1 cup whole wheat breadcrumbs

- 1/4 cup grated Parmesan cheese

- 1 teaspoon dried oregano

- 1 teaspoon dried basil

- 1/2 teaspoon garlic powder

- Salt and pepper to taste

- 2 large eggs, beaten

- 2 cups marinara sauce (store-bought or homemade)

- 1 cup shredded mozzarella cheese

- Fresh basil leaves for garnish

Preparation:

1. Preheat the oven to 400°F (200°C). Grease a baking sheet.

2. In a shallow dish, mix whole wheat breadcrumbs, grated Parmesan cheese,

dried oregano, dried basil, garlic powder, salt, and pepper.

3. Dip each eggplant round into the beaten eggs, then coat it with the breadcrumb mixture, pressing down gently to adhere the breadcrumbs to the eggplant.

4. Place the coated eggplant rounds on the prepared baking sheet.

5. Bake the eggplant in the preheated oven for about 15-20 minutes or until the eggplant is tender and the breadcrumbs are golden and crispy.

6. Remove the baked eggplant from the oven and reduce the oven temperature to 375°F (190°C).

7. In a baking dish, spread a thin layer of marinara sauce on the bottom.

8. Arrange a layer of baked eggplant rounds over the sauce.

9. Top the eggplant with more marinara sauce and shredded mozzarella cheese.

10. Repeat the layers until all the eggplant is used, finishing with a layer of sauce and cheese on top.

11. Bake the eggplant Parmesan in the reduced oven temperature for about 20-25 minutes or until the cheese is melted and bubbly.

12. Garnish with fresh basil leaves before serving this delicious and comforting dinner.

Day 26

Breakfast - Breakfast Burrito:

Ingredients:

- 2 large whole grain tortillas

- 4 large eggs, scrambled

- 1 cup black beans, drained and rinsed

- 1 cup diced tomatoes

- 1/2 cup diced red onion

- 1/2 cup shredded cheddar cheese

- 1 tablespoon olive oil

- Salt and pepper to taste

- Fresh cilantro for garnish

- Salsa or hot sauce (optional)

Preparation:

1. In a skillet, heat olive oil over medium heat.

2. Add diced red onion and sauté for about 2-3 minutes until they become translucent.

3. Add diced tomatoes and black beans to the skillet. Cook for another 2 minutes until the tomatoes are slightly softened.

4. Push the vegetable mixture to one side of the skillet and pour beaten eggs into the empty space.

5. Scramble the eggs until they are cooked through and set.

6. Combine the scrambled eggs with the sautéed vegetables in the skillet. Season with salt and pepper to taste.

7. Warm the whole grain tortillas in a separate skillet or microwave until they are pliable.

8. Place half of the scrambled eggs and vegetable mixture onto each tortilla.

9. Sprinkle shredded cheddar cheese over the filling.

10. Roll up the tortillas to form breakfast burritos.

11. Garnish with fresh cilantro and serve with salsa or hot sauce on the side, if desired.

Lunch - Mediterranean Chickpea Salad:

Ingredients:

- 1 can (15 ounces) chickpeas, drained and rinsed
- 1 cup diced cucumber
- 1 cup cherry tomatoes, halved
- 1/2 cup diced red onion
- 1/4 cup sliced Kalamata olives
- 1/4 cup crumbled feta cheese
- 2 tablespoons chopped fresh parsley
- 2 tablespoons lemon juice
- 2 tablespoons extra-virgin olive oil

- 1 teaspoon dried oregano

- Salt and pepper to taste

Preparation:

1. In a large bowl, combine chickpeas, diced cucumber, halved cherry tomatoes, diced red onion, sliced Kalamata olives, crumbled feta cheese, and chopped fresh parsley.

2. In a separate small bowl, whisk together lemon juice, extra-virgin olive oil, dried oregano, salt, and pepper to create the dressing.

3. Pour the dressing over the chickpea salad and toss everything together to coat.

4. Serve this refreshing and protein-rich Mediterranean chickpea salad for a light and satisfying lunch.

Dinner - Beef and Vegetable Stir-Fry:

Ingredients:

- 1 pound beef sirloin or flank steak, thinly sliced
- 2 tablespoons low-sodium soy sauce
- 2 tablespoons oyster sauce
- 1 tablespoon hoisin sauce (optional)
- 1 tablespoon cornstarch
- 2 tablespoons vegetable oil
- 2 cups broccoli florets
- 1 cup sliced bell peppers (any color)
- 1 cup sliced carrots
- 1 cup sliced mushrooms
- 2 cloves garlic, minced
- 1 tablespoon grated ginger
- 2 tablespoons chopped green onions (scallions)
- Sesame seeds for garnish

Preparation:

1. In a bowl, mix thinly sliced beef with low-sodium soy sauce, oyster sauce, hoisin sauce (if using), and cornstarch. Toss until the beef is evenly coated with the sauce.

2. In a large skillet or wok, heat vegetable oil over medium-high heat.

3. Add minced garlic and grated ginger to the skillet. Sauté for about 30 seconds until fragrant.

4. Add the marinated beef to the skillet and stir-fry for about 3-4 minutes until the beef is browned and cooked to your desired level of doneness.

5. Remove the cooked beef from the skillet and set aside.

6. In the same skillet, add more oil if needed, then add broccoli florets, sliced

bell peppers, sliced carrots, and sliced mushrooms. Stir-fry the vegetables for about 4-5 minutes until they become slightly tender but still crisp.

7. Return the cooked beef to the skillet with the vegetables.

8. Pour any remaining sauce from the marinated beef over the stir-fry and toss everything together to combine.

9. Stir-fry for another minute or two until the beef and vegetables are coated with the sauce and everything is heated through.

10. Sprinkle chopped green onions and sesame seeds over the beef and vegetable stir-fry for added flavor and garnish.

11. Serve this savory and satisfying beef and vegetable stir-fry over cooked brown rice or noodles for a delicious and hearty dinner.

Day 27

Breakfast - Banana Walnut Muffins:

Ingredients:
- 1 1/2 cups whole wheat flour
- 1/2 cup rolled oats
- 1/2 cup chopped walnuts
- 2 ripe bananas, mashed
- 1/2 cup unsweetened applesauce
- 1/4 cup honey or maple syrup
- 1/4 cup unsweetened almond milk (or any milk of choice)
- 1 large egg
- 1 teaspoon baking powder
- 1/2 teaspoon baking soda
- 1/2 teaspoon ground cinnamon
- 1/4 teaspoon salt

Preparation:

1. Preheat the oven to 350°F (175°C). Grease or line a muffin tin with paper liners.

2. In a large bowl, combine whole wheat flour, rolled oats, chopped walnuts, baking powder, baking soda, ground cinnamon, and salt.

3. In a separate bowl, mix mashed bananas, unsweetened applesauce, honey or maple syrup, unsweetened almond milk, and the egg until well combined.

4. Pour the wet ingredients into the dry ingredients and stir until just combined. Do not overmix.

5. Spoon the muffin batter into the prepared muffin tin, filling each cup about 2/3 full.

6. Bake the muffins in the preheated oven for about 18-20 minutes or until a toothpick

inserted into the center of a muffin comes out clean.

7. Remove the muffins from the oven and let them cool in the muffin tin for a few minutes before transferring them to a wire rack to cool completely.

8. Enjoy these delicious and wholesome banana walnut muffins for a satisfying breakfast or snack.

Lunch - Quinoa Salad with Roasted Vegetables:

Ingredients:

- 1 cup cooked quinoa (follow package instructions)
- 1 cup cherry tomatoes, halved
- 1 cup diced cucumbers
- 1/2 cup diced red onion
- 1/4 cup crumbled feta cheese

- 2 tablespoons chopped fresh parsley

- 2 tablespoons olive oil

- 1 tablespoon red wine vinegar

- 1 teaspoon dried oregano

- Salt and pepper to taste

For Roasted Vegetables:

- 2 cups mixed vegetables (bell peppers, zucchini, eggplant, etc.), cut into bite-sized pieces
- 2 tablespoons olive oil
- 1 teaspoon dried thyme
- Salt and pepper to taste

Preparation:

1. Preheat the oven to 425°F (220°C). Line a baking sheet with parchment paper.
2. In a bowl, toss the mixed vegetables with olive oil, dried thyme, salt, and pepper until well coated.
3. Spread the vegetables in a single layer on the prepared baking sheet.
4. Roast the vegetables in the preheated oven for about 20-25 minutes or until they are tender and slightly caramelized.
5. In a large bowl, combine cooked quinoa, halved cherry tomatoes, diced cucumbers,

diced red onion, crumbled feta cheese, and chopped fresh parsley.

6. In a separate small bowl, whisk together olive oil, red wine vinegar, dried oregano, salt, and pepper to create the dressing.

7. Pour the dressing over the quinoa salad and toss everything together to coat.

8. Add the roasted vegetables to the quinoa salad and gently toss to combine.

9. Serve this hearty and flavorful quinoa salad with roasted vegetables for a satisfying and nutritious lunch.

Dinner - Lemon Herb Baked Salmon:

Ingredients:

- 2 salmon fillets (about 6 ounces each)

- 2 tablespoons olive oil

- Zest and juice of 1 lemon

- 2 cloves garlic, minced

- 1 tablespoon chopped fresh dill

- 1 tablespoon chopped fresh parsley

- Salt and pepper to taste

Preparation:

1. Preheat the oven to 400°F (200°C). Grease a baking dish.

2. Place the salmon fillets in the prepared baking dish.

3. In a bowl, mix olive oil, lemon zest, lemon juice, minced garlic, chopped fresh

dill, chopped fresh parsley, salt, and pepper to create the marinade.

4. Pour the marinade over the salmon fillets, coating them evenly.

5. Bake the salmon in the preheated oven for about 12-15 minutes or until the fish is fully cooked and flakes easily with a fork.

6. Remove the baked salmon from the oven and let it rest for a few minutes before serving.

7. Serve this lemon herb baked salmon with your choice of side dishes, such as roasted vegetables or a green salad, for a delicious and healthy dinner.

Day 28

Breakfast - Chia Seed Yogurt Parfait:

Ingredients:

- 1/4 cup chia seeds
- 1 cup plain Greek yogurt
- 1 tablespoon honey or maple syrup (optional, for added sweetness)
- 1 cup mixed fresh berries (blueberries, strawberries, raspberries)
- 2 tablespoons granola
- Fresh mint leaves for garnish

Preparation:

1. In a bowl, mix chia seeds with plain Greek yogurt.

2. If desired, add honey or maple syrup to the yogurt mixture for added sweetness.

3. Cover the bowl and refrigerate for at least 4 hours or overnight to allow the chia seeds to absorb the yogurt and form a pudding-like consistency.

4. Before serving, give the chia seed yogurt parfait a good stir.

5. Layer the chia seed yogurt mixture with mixed fresh berries and granola in a glass or a bowl.

6. Garnish with fresh mint leaves before enjoying this creamy and nutrient-packed breakfast.

Lunch - Quinoa Stuffed Bell Peppers with Feta:

Ingredients:

- 2 large bell peppers (any color), halved and seeds removed

- 1 cup cooked quinoa (follow package instructions)

- 1 cup chopped spinach

- 1/2 cup crumbled feta cheese

- 1/4 cup diced red onion

- 2 tablespoons chopped fresh dill

- 1 tablespoon olive oil

- 1 tablespoon fresh lemon juice

- Salt and pepper to taste

Preparation:

1. Preheat the oven to 375°F (190°C). Grease a baking dish.

2. In a large bowl, combine cooked quinoa, chopped spinach, crumbled feta cheese,

diced red onion, chopped fresh dill, olive oil, fresh lemon juice, salt, and pepper.

3. Stuff the halved bell peppers with the quinoa and feta mixture, pressing down gently to fill each pepper evenly.

4. Place the stuffed bell peppers in the prepared baking dish.

5. Cover the baking dish with foil and bake in the preheated oven for about 20-25 minutes or until the bell peppers are tender.

6. Remove the foil from the baking dish and continue baking the stuffed bell peppers for an additional 5-10 minutes, or until the tops are slightly browned.

7. Once the bell peppers are cooked to your liking, remove them from the oven and let them cool slightly before serving.

8. Serve these flavorful and colorful quinoa stuffed bell peppers with feta as a wholesome and satisfying lunch.

Dinner - Shrimp and Asparagus Stir-Fry:

Ingredients:

- 1 pound large shrimp, peeled and deveined

- 1 bunch asparagus, trimmed and cut into bite-sized pieces

- 1 red bell pepper, sliced

- 2 cloves garlic, minced

- 1 tablespoon grated ginger

- 2 tablespoons low-sodium soy sauce

- 1 tablespoon oyster sauce

- 1 tablespoon sesame oil

- 2 tablespoons vegetable oil

- 2 tablespoons chopped green onions (scallions)

- Sesame seeds for garnish

Preparation:

1. In a bowl, mix shrimp with low-sodium soy sauce and oyster sauce. Toss until the shrimp is evenly coated with the sauce.

2. In a large skillet or wok, heat vegetable oil over medium-high heat.

3. Add minced garlic and grated ginger to the skillet. Sauté for about 30 seconds until fragrant.

4. Add sliced red bell pepper and asparagus pieces to the skillet. Stir-fry the vegetables for about 3-4 minutes until they become slightly tender but still crisp.

5. Push the vegetables to one side of the skillet and add the marinated shrimp to the empty space.

6. Stir-fry the shrimp for about 2-3 minutes on each side until they turn pink and are cooked through.

7. Combine the cooked shrimp with the sautéed vegetables in the skillet. Drizzle

sesame oil over the stir-fry and toss everything together to combine.

8. Stir-fry for another minute or two until the shrimp and vegetables are evenly coated with the sauce.

9. Sprinkle chopped green onions and sesame seeds over the shrimp and asparagus stir-fry for added flavor and garnish.

10. Serve this delicious and light shrimp and asparagus stir-fry over cooked brown rice or noodles for a quick and satisfying dinner.

Day 29

Breakfast - Veggie Omelette:

Ingredients:

- 4 large eggs

- 1/4 cup diced bell peppers (any color)

- 1/4 cup diced tomatoes

- 1/4 cup chopped spinach

- 1/4 cup diced onions

- 1/4 cup shredded cheddar cheese

- 1 tablespoon olive oil

- Salt and pepper to taste

- Fresh herbs (such as parsley or chives) for garnish

Preparation:

1. In a bowl, beat the eggs until well combined. Season with salt and pepper.

2. In a skillet, heat olive oil over medium heat.

3. Add diced onions and sauté for about 2-3 minutes until they become translucent.

4. Add diced bell peppers, diced tomatoes, and chopped spinach to the skillet. Sauté the vegetables for another 2-3 minutes until they are slightly tender.

5. Pour the beaten eggs over the sautéed vegetables in the skillet.

6. Let the eggs cook undisturbed for a minute or two until the edges start to set.

7. Sprinkle shredded cheddar cheese over one-half of the omelette.

8. Carefully fold the other half of the omelette over the cheese side, creating a half-moon shape.

9. Cook the omelette for another minute or two until the cheese is melted and the eggs are fully cooked.

10. Slide the veggie omelette onto a plate and garnish with fresh herbs before serving this hearty and protein-rich breakfast.

Lunch - Chicken Avocado Wrap:

Ingredients:

- 2 large whole wheat tortillas

- 1 cup cooked and shredded chicken (rotisserie chicken works well)

- 1 ripe avocado, sliced

- 1/2 cup mixed salad greens (such as lettuce or spinach)

- 1/4 cup diced tomatoes

- 2 tablespoons plain Greek yogurt or sour cream

- 1 tablespoon fresh lime juice

- Salt and pepper to taste

Preparation:

1. In a small bowl, mix plain Greek yogurt or sour cream with fresh lime juice. Season

with salt and pepper to create a creamy dressing.

2. Lay the whole wheat tortillas flat on a clean surface.

3. Divide the shredded chicken evenly between the two tortillas, placing it in the center of each.

4. Top the chicken with sliced avocado, mixed salad greens, and diced tomatoes.

5. Drizzle the creamy dressing over the fillings in each tortilla.

6. Fold the sides of the tortillas in, then roll them up tightly to form wraps.

7. Slice the wraps in half if desired and secure them with toothpicks.

8. Serve these delicious and satisfying chicken avocado wraps for a quick and portable lunch.

Dinner - Vegetarian Pad Thai:

Ingredients:

- 8 ounces rice noodles

- 1 cup cubed tofu

- 1 cup broccoli florets

- 1/2 cup shredded carrots

- 1/2 cup sliced bell peppers (any color)

- 1/4 cup sliced green onions (scallions)

- 2 cloves garlic, minced

- 2 tablespoons vegetable oil

- 2 tablespoons soy sauce

- 2 tablespoons tamarind paste

- 1 tablespoon brown sugar

- 1 tablespoon lime juice

- 1 tablespoon chopped peanuts

- Fresh cilantro for garnish

Preparation:

1. Cook the rice noodles according to the package instructions. Drain and set aside.

2. In a large skillet or wok, heat vegetable oil over medium-high heat.

3. Add minced garlic and cubed tofu to the skillet. Sauté the tofu until it becomes slightly crispy and golden.

4. Add broccoli florets, shredded carrots, and sliced bell peppers to the skillet. Stir-fry the vegetables for about 3-4 minutes until they are slightly tender but still crisp.

5. In a small bowl, whisk together soy sauce, tamarind paste, brown sugar, and lime juice to create the Pad Thai sauce.

6. Pour the sauce over the vegetables and tofu in the skillet. Toss everything together to coat.

7. Add the cooked rice noodles to the skillet and stir-fry everything together for another minute or two until the noodles are well coated with the sauce.

8. Sprinkle sliced green onions and chopped peanuts over the Pad Thai for added flavor and garnish.

9. Serve this flavorful and satisfying vegetarian Pad Thai for a delicious and wholesome dinner.

Day 30

Breakfast - Smoothie Bowl:

Ingredients:

- 1 cup frozen mixed berries (blueberries, strawberries, raspberries)
- 1 ripe banana
- 1 cup plain Greek yogurt
- 1/2 cup unsweetened almond milk (or any milk of choice)
- 1 tablespoon honey or maple syrup (optional, for added sweetness)
- Toppings: sliced fresh fruit, granola, chia seeds, shredded coconut

Preparation:

1. In a blender, combine frozen mixed berries, ripe banana, plain Greek yogurt, and unsweetened almond milk.

2. Blend until the mixture is smooth and creamy.

3. If desired, add honey or maple syrup to the smoothie mixture for added sweetness.

4. Pour the smoothie into a bowl.

5. Top the smoothie with sliced fresh fruit, granola, chia seeds, and shredded coconut for a delicious and nutrient-packed breakfast.

6. Enjoy the smoothie bowl with a spoon for a refreshing and satisfying start to your day.

Lunch - Spinach and Feta Stuffed Chicken Breast:

Ingredients:

- 2 boneless, skinless chicken breasts

- 1 cup chopped spinach

- 1/2 cup crumbled feta cheese

- 1 tablespoon olive oil

- 1 teaspoon dried oregano

- Salt and pepper to taste

Preparation:

1. Preheat the oven to 375°F (190°C). Grease a baking dish.

2. Using a sharp knife, create a pocket in each chicken breast by cutting a slit horizontally into the thickest part of the meat, being careful not to cut all the way through.

3. In a bowl, mix chopped spinach, crumbled feta cheese, olive oil, dried oregano, salt, and pepper.

4. Stuff each chicken breast with the spinach and feta mixture, pressing down gently to fill each pocket evenly.

5. Place the stuffed chicken breasts in the prepared baking dish.

6. Bake the chicken in the preheated oven for about 25-30 minutes or until the chicken is fully cooked and reaches an internal temperature of 165°F (74°C).

7. Remove the stuffed chicken breasts from the oven and let them rest for a few minutes before slicing.

8. Serve the spinach and feta stuffed chicken breast with a side salad or your choice of roasted vegetables for a tasty and protein-packed lunch.

Dinner - Mushroom and Spinach Pasta:

Ingredients:

- 8 ounces whole wheat or regular pasta of your choice
- 2 cups sliced mushrooms (any variety)
- 2 cups chopped spinach
- 2 cloves garlic, minced
- 1/4 cup grated Parmesan cheese
- 2 tablespoons olive oil
- 1 tablespoon unsalted butter (optional, for added richness)
- Salt and pepper to taste
- Fresh parsley for garnish

Preparation:

1. Cook the pasta according to the package instructions. Drain and set aside.

2. In a large skillet, heat olive oil over medium heat.

3. Add minced garlic to the skillet and sauté for about 30 seconds until fragrant.

4. Add sliced mushrooms to the skillet and cook for about 5 minutes until they are tender and slightly browned.

5. Stir in the chopped spinach and cook for another 2 minutes until the spinach wilts.

6. If desired, stir in unsalted butter for added richness to the sauce.

7. Add the cooked pasta to the skillet and toss everything together to combine.

8. Sprinkle grated Parmesan cheese over the pasta and toss again until the cheese is melted and coats the pasta.

9. Season with salt and pepper to taste.

10. Garnish the mushroom and spinach pasta with fresh parsley before serving this comforting and flavorful dinner.

Snack - Apple Slices with Almond Butter:

Ingredients:

- 1 apple, sliced

- 2 tablespoons almond butter

Preparation:

1. Wash the apple and cut it into slices.

2. Serve the apple slices with almond butter on the side for dipping.

3. Enjoy this simple and nutritious snack for a burst of energy and a satisfying treat.

Congratulations on completing your 30-day meal plan! I hope you find these recipes delicious and enjoyable. If you have any dietary preferences or specific requests for future meal plans, feel free to let me know. Happy cooking and bon appétit!

CONCLUSION

As we come to the final pages of this diabetes cookbook, we find ourselves filled with a sense of gratitude and wonder at the incredible journey we've taken together. This culinary adventure has been so much more than just a collection of recipes – it has been a celebration of resilience, the triumph of the human spirit, and the transformative power of stories.

Throughout this cookbook, we have delved into the lives of remarkable individuals who have faced the challenges of diabetes with unwavering determination. Their stories have touched our hearts, reminding us of the strength that lies within us all. As we cooked their cherished recipes, we connected with their experiences, finding inspiration in their courage and perseverance.

We've learned that the kitchen can be a place of healing and empowerment, where ingredients can be transformed into nourishing meals that sustain both body and soul. Mindful cooking has become a way of life, and each recipe carries with it the love and care with which it was prepared.

In these pages, we have celebrated the diverse flavors and cultures that come together to create a harmonious symphony of taste. From comforting classics to bold innovations, we have embraced the richness of culinary exploration while keeping health at the forefront.

Beyond the tangible nourishment, this cookbook has shown us the intangible power of storytelling. The narratives shared here have united us, fostering empathy and understanding among the community. We've discovered that stories can be a bridge that connects us, erasing barriers and building a sense of belonging.

As we close this chapter, let us carry forward the spirit of Isabella and the countless others who have left an indelible mark on these pages. Let this cookbook be more than just a recipe guide on your shelf – let it be a constant reminder that life's challenges can be met with courage, hope, and love. Embrace the journey, savor the flavors, and cherish the stories that make life truly remarkable.

Above all, may this cookbook be a beacon of hope for those living with diabetes, a reminder that they are not alone on their path. Together, we can navigate the complexities of diabetes and find joy in the art of cooking, knowing that every meal we prepare is a testament to our resilience and a celebration of life's vibrant tapestry.

As we bid farewell to this culinary voyage, remember that every dish you create carries a story of its own – a story that adds depth and meaning to the food on your plate. So, embrace the joy of cooking, the power of storytelling, and the magic that lies within each one of us. Bon appétit and bon voyage on your continued journey of living well and thriving with diabetes.

Happy Cooking!!!

www.ingramcontent.com/pod-product-compliance
Lightning Source LLC
Chambersburg PA
CBHW070940250726

48663CB00001B/9